SAGE was founded in 1965 by Sara Miller McCune to support the dissemination of usable knowledge by publishing innovative and high-quality research and teaching content. Today, we publish over 900 journals, including those of more than 400 learned societies, more than 800 new books per year, and a growing range of library products including archives, data, case studies, reports, and video. SAGE remains majority-owned by our founder, and after Sara's lifetime will become owned by a charitable trust that secures our continued independence.

Los Angeles | London | New Delhi | Singapore | Washington DC | Melbourne

DISABILITY and CARE WORK

Thank you for choosing a SAGE product!
If you have any comment, observation or feedback,
I would like to personally hear from you.

Please write to me at **contactceo@sagepub.in**

Vivek Mehra, Managing Director and CEO, SAGE India.

Bulk Sales

SAGE India offers special discounts
for purchase of books in bulk.
We also make available special imprints
and excerpts from our books on demand.

For orders and enquiries, write to us at

Marketing Department
SAGE Publications India Pvt Ltd
B1/I-1, Mohan Cooperative Industrial Area
Mathura Road, Post Bag 7
New Delhi 110044, India

E-mail us at **marketing@sagepub.in**

Get to know more about SAGE
Be invited to SAGE events, get on our mailing list.
Write today to **marketing@sagepub.in**

This book is also available as an e-book.

DISABILITY and CARE WORK

State, Society and Invisible Lives

UPALI CHAKRAVARTI

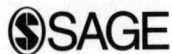

Los Angeles | London | New Delhi
Singapore | Washington DC | Melbourne

Copyright © Upali Chakravarti, 2018

All rights reserved. No part of this book may be reproduced or utilised in any form or by any means, electronic or mechanical, including photocopying, recording, or by any information storage or retrieval system, without permission in writing from the publisher.

First published in 2018 by

SAGE Publications India Pvt Ltd
B1/I-1 Mohan Cooperative Industrial Area
Mathura Road, New Delhi 110 044, India
www.sagepub.in

SAGE Publications Inc
2455 Teller Road
Thousand Oaks, California 91320, USA

SAGE Publications Ltd
1 Oliver's Yard, 55 City Road
London EC1Y 1SP, United Kingdom

SAGE Publications Asia-Pacific Pte Ltd
3 Church Street
#10-04 Samsung Hub
Singapore 049483

Published by Vivek Mehra for SAGE Publications India Pvt Ltd, typeset in 10.5/13 pts Berkeley by Zaza Eunice, Hosur, Tamil Nadu, India and printed at Chaman Enterprises, New Delhi.

Library of Congress Cataloging-in-Publication Data

Name: Chakravarti, Upali, author.
Title: Disability and care work: state, society and invisible lives/Upali Chakravarti.
Description: New Delhi, India: SAGE Publications India, 2018. | Includes bibliographical references and index.
Identifiers: LCCN 2018031089 | ISBN 9789352807741 (hbk: alk. paper) | ISBN 9789352807765 (ebook) | ISBN 9789352807758 (epub 2.0)
Subjects: LCSH: People with disabilities—Care. | People with disabilities—Social conditions. | Disabilities—Social aspects.
Classification: LCC HV1568 .C43 2018 | DDC 362.4/048—dc23 LC record available at https://lccn.loc.gov/2018031089

ISBN: 978-93-528-0774-1 (HB)

SAGE Team: Rajesh Dey, Guneet Kaur, Syeda Aina Rahat Ali and Ritu Chopra

CONTENTS

List of Abbreviations vii
Preface ix
Acknowledgements xiii

Part 1

    Chapter 1 Introduction 3
    Chapter 2 Framing Disability 13

Part 2

    Chapter 3 Making Sense of the Narratives I: Experiencing Disability—Inter-class Dimensions 31

    Chapter 4 Making Sense of the Narratives II: Living with Disability 88

    Chapter 5 Making Sense of the Narratives III: Invisible Work, Invisible Women—Caring for the Disabled 119

Part 3

    Chapter 6 State, Society and Disability in India 145
    Chapter 7 The Welfare State as Paternalistic Caregiver 169

Chapter 8	Conclusion: The Moral and Political Economy of Disability and Suffering	189

Appendix 209
Bibliography 210
Index 216
About the Author 220

LIST OF ABBREVIATIONS

AADI	Action for Ability Development and Inclusion
ADAPT	Able Disabled All People Together
AIIMS	All India Institute of Medical Sciences
ART	assisted reproductive technologies
CAPART	Council for Advancement of People's Action and Rural Technology
CBR	community-based rehabilitation
CP	cerebral palsy
CRPD	Convention on the Rights of Persons with Disabilities
CSE	*Centre for Special Education*
DPEP	District Primary Education Programme
DRG	Disability Rights Group
ICDS	Integrated Child Development Services
ICIDH	*International Classification of Impairments, Disabilities and Handicaps*
NCPEDP	National Centre for Promotion of Employment for Disabled Persons
NCR	National Capital Region
NHS	national health service
NSS	National Sample Survey
PHC	primary health care

SHGs	self-help groups
SSNI	Spastics Society of Northern India
TIE	Together in Education
VS	Vidya Sagar

PREFACE

When I was a student of a special education course in New Delhi during the 1990s, every morning I would take a bus from Kashmere Gate to Vasant Vihar, where the institution that conducted the course was located. I soon made friends with another young woman who was a regular on the bus, and we fell to chatting as it often happens in buses. We talked about many things; soon she knew that I was training to be a special educator for children with disabilities, and she, in turn, shared information about her interests and her family. Despite knowing what my area of work was going to be, many months passed us by before she told me about her sister who was disabled. It was only after this closely guarded secret was finally revealed that our everyday conversations became interspersed with little details about her sister, and that made me think about the burdens that families of the disabled carry with them at all times but cannot share with others most of the time.

Perhaps this encounter in the bus was the trigger that expanded my interest beyond people with disabilities, to their families. Later in my career as someone who worked in the areas of psychology, health and inclusive education for over a decade, I met a number of people working in similar fields as well as others including people with psychological conditions, health issues and a child with disability, who shared their experiences with me. Listening to their stories and interacting with them, sometimes just as a co-passenger in a bus, or on a more long-term basis as a therapist or as an educator, brought me to the realisation that caring and suffering are among the two most important aspects of any person's life. I then realised that these two aspects of the 'lived' experience of people are very often underestimated in many different areas of study and work that I have encountered.

Caring and suffering could even be termed as the unmet needs of people that have not been addressed adequately by social science researchers. Both caring and suffering have been regarded as an individual experience, largely determined by individual circumstances except in certain situations, involving larger groups of people in times of war, genocide and famine. In discussions around health, caring and suffering are also individualised with regard to the solutions offered. It is also significant that when an attempt is made to put them in a context, caring and suffering have been linked to culture more often than to the political economy. We, therefore, have only a partial understanding of both phenomena. There is, thus, a need to contextualise caring and suffering with regard to the political economy, and also to the lived experiences of people, as well as the ethical choices they make to surmount the difficult situations they face.

Concerns such as these are beginning to be reflected in social science and medical research in recent years (Farmer 1997; Russell 1999; Turnbull 2000). Within the area of disability, over the past two decades, the field of disability studies has experienced growth and expansion in the understanding of wider issues concerned with disability. The concerns are no longer just limited to experiences of personal heroism in overcoming disability that dominated early writings on disability. Instead, these concerns now seek to address larger issues in the context of the political economy, and the framework of rights. These developments and recent research have opened up the possibility of examining disability, caring, suffering and the ethical choices associated with them.

In brief, I chose to study caring and suffering in the context of disability because whether one studies ill health, well-being, welfare, gender, state or society, or the margins of society, disability has remained a relatively unexplored field in India. It is as if the 'stigma' of disability that throws a cloak of invisibility over the disabled members of a society has, in turn, made disability invisible within the social sciences as well. Fortunately, in the last decade or so, disability issues have gained prominence. As a result, in various international and global forums and reports, disability issues have come to be included. For instance, while the *Human Development Reports* of the 1990s did not mention the term disability, during the decade of the 2000s, the United Nations had to come out with the Convention on the Rights of Persons with Disabilities (CRPD). Beyond this, the most recent example is the World Health Organization–World Bank *World Report on Disability* (2011).

However, there are very few studies dealing with the low priority given to disability in conceptualising the public health needs of a society (Allen 1998; Jones 1998; Pardo 2000). Despite the claim that the goal of alleviating suffering is integral to public health, it has failed to include disability within its purview. Although the data indicates that a small proportion of the population is disabled, this small proportion constitutes a large minority, and disability can afflict anyone at any time (Census of India 1981; NSSO 1981). Closer to home, public health is defined as the organised effort of the community to deal with disease prevention, cure and rehabilitation. This definition seems to indicate that public health deals with not only the individual but also the community within which the person resides. On the other hand, public health departments and courses rarely include disability in India. Therefore, to rectify this omission, I was drawn towards a field of research that would bring disability, caregiving and social suffering together. The appeal of this research made sense to me, given my background specialising in developmental psychology, and subsequent training and work as a special educator in the field of special education, and finally the impressions I gained through my interactions with a teacher who had a disability, when I was an undergraduate student.

ACKNOWLEDGEMENTS

I would like to acknowledge my deep gratitude to all those who guided, supported and encouraged me to undertake this research in the field of disability. I thank the parents and children who gave of themselves most generously, and I hope that this work will provide, at least in a small measure, an insight into their lives and many others placed in similar situations so that their voices are heard and their experiences are validated. I am extremely grateful for the enthusiastic encouragement shown to me by Dr Rama V. Baru, who supervised my thesis; Dr Anita Ghai, who taught me as an undergraduate student; and Ms Poonam Natarajan, whom I met in Chennai when I was doing my research work, on undertaking this study. I am also grateful to the staff at Action for Ability Development and Inclusion, New Delhi, and Vidya Sagar, Chennai, for helping me to access the families; and to the professionals and activists involved in the field of disability whom I interviewed for this work. I am also extremely grateful to Ms Anshu Dogra for her invaluable and timely support in helping me to keep to my deadlines in preparing this manuscript and to the SAGE team for facilitating the publication of this book. I also thank my friends, who are too numerous to name, for their solidarity and friendship over the years. And, finally, I thank my family for the generous support that they extended throughout my journey, beginning with the years of research work and finally in the completion of the book.

PART 1

Introduction

A review of the literature on the subject of disability shows that the issue of disability and the experiences of persons with disabilities have been given scant consideration in the academic arena. The two disciplines that have worked in the area of disability are medicine and psychology. However, in both disciplines, the predominant context of reference is medical. Further, psychology not only views disability as a 'problem' but also emphasises the need for 'adjustment' by the person with disability to the 'normal' environment. None of the other academic disciplines, such as sociology, history, political science, anthropology and social policy, have developed theories or understandings other than basing studies in a medical context. The focal points of discussion within the disciplines, particularly medical sociology and anthropology, often get restricted to distinguishing illness, health and disability, again indicating a strong leaning towards the medical model of disability.

Another crucial aspect that dominates the understanding of disability is the highly individualised nature attributed to the issue of disability. Apart from the medical condition, the approach to disability is that it is viewed as an individual problem that must be handled or dealt with at the individual level. Such a view relegates the issue of disability outside the purview of studies that try to understand the nature of social relations in the relevant field of enquiry.

These two approaches to disability have led many disability rights activists and scholars to identify the real causes for the exclusion of persons with disabilities from the larger studies of society, politics and economics. Dominant views of disability, as individual and medical problems, have been challenged mostly by persons with disabilities themselves. The restrictions placed on the abilities and lives of persons with disabilities due to these narrow views have sown the first seeds of the development of disability studies as a discipline.

This book explores the experience of disability and its consequences on the family and community vis-à-vis suffering. It focuses on the social context of caring and examines the problem of who actually bears the consequences of caregiving in the absence of adequate institutional and state support.

It is well recognised that for any condition, there are preventive, curative, promotive and palliative aspects. Thus, caring is an important component of any health system and is not just the need of a person or family. The concept of caring includes emotional and rehabilitative aspects. An interdisciplinary perspective on public health views the curative and rehabilitative aspects as ongoing processes. However, caregiving is not just about nursing. In chronic lifelong conditions, it involves social, economic and emotional aspects as well. With increasing de-institutionalisation, and the state's rapid withdrawal from the health and welfare sectors even in the developed countries, along with the limitations of the biomedical approach, caring is increasingly falling upon the family, and within the family upon women, especially in the case of persons with disabilities and the old.

Even though public health has had a dominant biomedical presence, by definition public health is an organised effort of the community to deal with the prevention of illness, cure and rehabilitation. Without underestimating the contribution of biomedicine, from this meaning of public health as an organised effort of the community, we can derive an expanded understanding of public health, which is that health is a collective creation of society. A consideration of causative factors opens up issues which fall within the wider social, economic and political spheres that may influence the perception and meanings of different health problems, and health behaviour.

This book attempts to explore another way of looking at the problem of not just disability but any chronic lifelong condition requiring caring, beginning with an understanding of the felt needs or expectations of the family and caregiver. As the condition of cerebral palsy (CP) involves lifelong caring, it is the special focus of this book.

On the basis of primary data and secondary literature, the book explores the level of state intervention vis-à-vis policies and legislation for the disabled, the extent of their implementation, and the success and failure achieved in meeting their aims.

The book also briefly traces the entry and role of the NGOs in the disability sector with regard to reasons for their entry into the sector, the type of services they provide, sections of the disabled they cater for, the extent to which they meet the needs of the disabled, and their role in advocacy for the disabled.

RATIONALE FOR CHOOSING FAMILIES OF PERSONS WITH CP

In my experience of working with children and adults with disabilities, I came across CP as one of the toughest disabilities to manage. It can be very mild; in this case, one cannot make out that a person has CP and he/she can go about his/her daily living without much of a problem. On the other hand, it can be so severe and profound due to its multiple manifestations that a person can be totally dependent. The extent of this dependency can be so extreme that the person needs help to do even a simple task such as lifting a finger or moving one's position while lying down. With regard to the data on disability, the National Sample Survey (NSS) shows that CP is the third highest cause of physical disability (the first two being burns and old age).

The book relies upon purposive sampling in order to study variations along income, age and condition. The two conditions of developmental CP taken were with mental retardation and without mental retardation. A sample of 37 families was taken from rural and urban settings. Three income categories were considered: those with incomes less than ₹3,000 per month; those with incomes between ₹3,000 and ₹15,000 per month; and those with incomes above ₹15,000 per month. The age group taken was 5 years to 30+ years. The sample of 37 families was taken from Action for Ability Development and Inclusion (AADI[1]), New Delhi (24 families), and Vidya Sagar (VS), Chennai (13 families). These two organisations were chosen because both have had links with the original Spastics Society of India, Mumbai (now ADAPT). They also have vast experience working in the field of disability, particularly with children and persons with CP and their families. The two organisations were a measure for any regional and cultural variations in the problem being studied. Another important reason was that VS has residential facilities, enabling young people to live away from home and pursue education/skill building which AADI does not have.

The core of the study explores the lived experience of the caregiver families and their life with the child or person with disability. The study comprises narratives collected from young people and members of their families, especially mothers, to explore variations along income, age and the condition of CP. These objectives were pursued through in-depth case studies generated by following a checklist of open-ended questions, with appropriate probes about the case histories of the individuals who have suffered the effects of CP. In addition, in-depth interviews had been used to elicit information from families, caregivers and other persons who had experienced disabilities, as well as from professionals and policy-makers.

Each of the interviews has been referred to as a narrative. Although the narratives have many issues and themes in common across different settings, each is unique in terms of the everyday experience of caring and living with disability. The subtle nuances of the situation come to the fore only from reading each narrative, for each says much more than just what is immediately visible, while becoming part of the analysis in this work. The richness of the narratives and

[1] http://aadi-india.org/our-journey/

the experiences contained therein form a part of the analysis of this work. Even though they are comparable to a bird's eye view of the individual situation in which the narrators are placed, the sum total is enormous if quantified through the multiplication of such experiences, for disability affects not just the individual but also each member of the family, across the country.

The interviews conducted in Delhi with families having a person with disability were in three groups—families residing in urban localities, families in the urban slums and families residing in semi-rural areas, mostly on the outskirts of Delhi but within the National Capital Region (NCR). The families in the urban localities and semi-rural areas were contacted through AADI, New Delhi. The families in the urban slums were contacted through an NGO working on a community-based project on disability and inclusive education in one of the biggest slum areas of Delhi.

The profile of the families residing in the urban localities belonged to the lower, middle and upper income groups. The families belonging to the semi-rural areas belonged to middle and lower income groups. The families living in the urban slums were understandably from the lower income group, and many were daily wage earners.

The families living in the urban and semi-rural areas had a long association with AADI. Some families' association coincided with the birth of their child and the inception of the organisation, which is an association of over three decades. Most of the families whose children had grown up were no longer coming to the organisation for reasons such as illness, difficulty in transportation, and mainly because they were not able to pursue any vocational skill development. However, some of the more 'able' ones had been enrolled in the vocational centre, and hence continued to come to the organisation on a regular basis.

On the other hand, the families in the urban slum area had very sporadic association with NGOs working in the area on the issue of disability. Most of the NGOs merely dealt with giving aids and appliances such as crutches or wheelchairs. This left out a big section of children who had disabilities other than those requiring crutches and wheelchairs. Hence, any sustained association the families had with an institution was with the hospitals they visited in the initial years after birth of their child with disability. However, thereafter, as the child grew older, even that contact discontinued and the person was homebound.

Another set of narratives is of families belonging to Chennai. They were contacted through the organisation called VS in Chennai. The families belonged to lower, middle and upper income groups. The parents ranged from businesspersons, other professionals and teachers to housemaids and ayahs. All the parents resided in Chennai city, though there were some who came from the outskirts of Chennai. Most of the children with disabilities were still attending different centres of the organisation. There were a few who were in an inclusive set-up such as a school but came to the centre for additional help. Many students were completing their education through the Open School, and the organisation was the space which provided them guidance and tuitions. Some of the students were involved in the vocational centre. The organisation even had provision to accommodate very severe cases of CP who required a bed. For instance, one girl had severe CP but had been trained in eye pointing and through that process, she was pursuing Open School learning. She used to come to the organisation to get help in her studies and take the examinations. Many of the mothers also spent time at the organisation either learning the tasks or helping the child learn the tasks. Some mothers were working in the organisation either as administrator, teacher, teacher trainer or ayah.

This book is organised in three parts: Part 1 frames the work in the context of the literature on the politics of disablement, the relationship between the political economy and disability policies, and locating the roots of social suffering. Part 2 comprises the analysis based on a set of narratives derived from the interviews I conducted with my informants. The families were contacted with the help of NGOs that have been working for a long time in the field of CP and disability issues. The NGOs in Delhi were AADI, also formerly known as the Spastics Society of Northern India (SSNI), and Together in Education

(TIE). The NGO contacted in Chennai was VS. The NGOs contacted the families, briefed them about my research work as per the synopsis I had submitted to the NGO and obtained their consent to give me an interview. The interviews were conducted in Hindi, English and Tamil. The transcriptions of the interviews conducted in Hindi and Tamil are translations which capture the essence of what the interviewees were discussing. The interviews vary in length, as the interviewees determined the course and duration of the interview: some were expansive in their answers and others were less so.

All the narratives highlight the direct experience of families of the person with disability, and the persons with disabilities themselves. The narratives draw attention to a range of issues such as caring, support for caring, living life with a disability and rights of persons with disabilities. This is the subject matter of the second part of the book. Part 2, thus, explores a range of issues that emerge from the similarities and differences of the experience of disability within families; institutional, cultural and social responses to disability; and with the provision of care to the disabled in the context of inter-class dimensions. The issue of caregiving is looked at conceptually and analytically, and is related to the ideologies of caring, theoretical perspectives on caring in the context of social justice and locating the roots of social suffering. Part 3 contextualises disability and caregiving with respect to the welfare state in theory and in practice, and the moral and political economy of disability and suffering.

DISABILITY, SOCIAL SUFFERING, CAREGIVING AND CP

In the past, disability was considered to be a purely medical or individualised concept. It is now largely accepted that this medical or individual model does not accurately describe the concept of disability. The model neglects highly important contextual factors that may greatly increase the functional limitations a person experiences. Maintaining medical or individual views of disability will, therefore, exclude people with disabilities in society. In order to include the perspectives of persons with disabilities in any process, the contextual factors that serve to exclude persons with disabilities need to be recognised and addressed.

Cerebral Palsy

'Cerebral palsy (CP) describes a group of permanent disorders of movement and posture, causing activity limitations that are attributed to non-progressive disturbances that occurred in the developing foetal or infant brain. The motor disorders of cerebral palsy are often accompanied by disturbances of sensation, perception, cognition, communication, and behaviour, by epilepsy, and by secondary musculoskeletal problems' (Cerebral Palsy Foundation[2]). However, even the combined use of terms that give the type and distribution of the movement disorder cannot give the whole story about any one individual as it gives no indication of the degree of severity of individual impairment. Nor does it give any information that refers to the presence or absence of any of the other handicaps that may accompany the motor disability—impairment of sight, hearing, speech and intellect—which occur in varying degrees of severity. It is also difficult to describe a typical person with CP. Each is different in some way from all the others, so much so that one is tempted to think that the cerebrally palsied have only their differences in common. This is borne out well in the individual narratives.

Care and Caregiving

Care is defined with reference to activities and relationships in connection with categories of vulnerable groups such as the very young, the ill and the elderly (Daly and Rake 2003). Care is both a social exigency and a form of interpersonal connection. It should be noted that although social policy is very important in determining the form and

[2] yourcpf.org

consequences of care, the political economy of care extends beyond public provisions. Even in societies in which the state provides many services, most care is provided informally in families and communities, and has invisible costs attached to it (Daly and Rake 2003).

Social Suffering

It is said that humankind's most fundamental beliefs are those that concern life, suffering and death. This leads to efforts to prolong life, alleviate suffering and prevent death. Such efforts bring into specific focus the roles of the medical sciences and health care strategies, and more generally a focus on the social, economic and political contexts of the development of these strategies.

This kind of grouping of human problems also defeats the categorisation of such issues, principally psychological, or medical, and therefore individual. Instead, it points to the invariably close link of personal problems with societal problems. It also reveals the interpersonal grounds of suffering; in other words, it reveals that suffering is a social experience. Social suffering is shared across high- and low-income societies, primarily affecting those who are desperately poor and powerless in such settings. Along with the fact that the subject of suffering cannot be examined as a single theme or a uniform experience, suffering is also profoundly social. Therefore, the instances giving rise to suffering are not merely a correlation but also a causal web in the global political economy (Kleinman, Das, and Lock 1997).

Suffering, as a social experience, in the Western tradition, lays emphasis on the subjective feelings of the afflicted individual, often viewed as isolated and forlorn. This is the dominant analytic paradigm for understanding suffering that results from serious chronic illness and disability. Framed this way, suffering becomes the pain, hurt, loss and search for meaning of a unique person, who alone must bear the deep burden of his/her troubles. Thus, the paradigmatic locus of suffering is the private space of the person with the problem.

However, Kleinman has argued that the locus of suffering should be in the inter-subjective space of interactions, especially with regard to families. Viewed this way, suffering is a mode of social experience. The point is not to minimise the seriousness of problems faced by the individual patients but rather to appreciate the importance that they and their families attribute to the interpersonal, relational locus of hardship among the family members. Therefore, suffering is as much the inter-subjective experience of parents, spouses, siblings and children as that of the sick person (Kleinman 1995, 163).

Appreciating the implications of the inter-subjective experience of suffering may begin with understanding its epistemological and moral basis. However, it eventually requires that we understand suffering as a different way of living through the illness in the social world. Even within the family, the social experience of suffering is not homogeneous, and it might even be divided. Some might even attempt to escape from it. On the other hand, time and again, mothers and wives cannot refuse but must endure. Accordingly, this work explores the various contexts in which the experience of disability may be understood.

Framing Disability

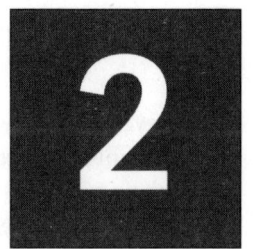

A number of general themes can be isolated in the review of literature on disability studies. These are: the debate on an appropriate definition of disability; the cultural context of the responses to disability; the ideological construction of disability, mainly the medicalisation and individualisation of disability; constructions of disabled identities from the perspective of psychology, social psychology, sociology, race and gender; and the social construction of disability, mainly from the political, economic and social policy perspectives.

DEFINING DISABILITY

Among the first issues to be taken up was the attempt to define disability in acceptable ways. The WHO's definition has generated considerable critical debate, primarily because the approach relies on medical definitions and uses a bio-physiological definition of 'normality'. Second, 'impairment' is identified as the cause of both 'disability' and 'handicap', thereby implying that the way to overcome 'disability' and social disadvantage is through appropriate medical and allied rehabilitative interventions. The criticism of the WHO's *International Classification of Impairments, Disabilities and Handicaps* (ICIDH) has led to bringing out a revised version after undergoing field testing which adopts a so-called 'bio-psychosocial' model that endeavours to synthesise the medical and social approaches to disability.

However, according to Barbara Harriss-White, no matter what the official definitions of disability, it is a relative term because cultures define their norms of 'being' and 'doing' in different ways (Harriss-White 1999, 135). In South Asia, for example, social deviancy is classified by many local people as a disability, as is being outcast from the caste system. Economically oppressive, socially tyrannical and politically disenfranchising forms of work such as child labour and bonded labour are sometimes considered to be disabling. Physical and mental disabilities, as recognised clinically and legally, may be considered as 'fitting' retribution for particular sins (in a past life), responsibility for which lies entirely with the individual.

Further, according to Harriss-White, as a form of deprivation, disability is intractably complex (Harriss-White 1999, 136). Yet the concept of 'disability' is a crude political label akin to that of being 'black'. Impairment forms a continuum from 'ability' to a range of kinds, combinations and intensities of incapacity. Medically, and sometimes for the purposes of legal claim, they are distinguished according to type and severity. The condition may be static or it may change progressively. That disability causes poverty is incontrovertible, but disability also affects the non-poor as well as the poor, and the social and economic costs of a given disability will differ according to social location, social or ethnic group, gender, age and economic status. Impairment may be ascribed a social stigma and may affect status as a citizen. Mortality may be heightened for social and economic rather than medical reasons. According to Harriss-White, the reasons for disability (disease, congenital causes, accident, war) can and do affect legal entitlement (Harriss-White 1999, 22–27).

CARING AND CAREGIVING: COMMUNITY, FAMILY AND GENDER

The organisation of caring in a given society is closely linked to the way in which the society organises different aspects of social relations. According to Gillian Dalley, under normal circumstances, within the context of the family, responsibility for fulfilling the caring and nurturing function in relation to the rearing of children and the servicing of adult family members falls upon women (Dalley 1988). Women are also expected in 'extra-normal' circumstances to care for the chronically dependent (the disabled and elderly) persons. In traditional societies, because there is relatively little specialised division of labour, caring gets absorbed into a collectivity if none of the functions is demarcated by a public–private dichotomy. According to Dalley (1988), what has been termed as the social construction of dependency is of a different order in such societies as compared to its capitalist construction. In the latter, those who cannot work (for wages) due to physical or mental impairment, or those who have passed beyond the age limit imposed by society on the end of working life, automatically become dependent either on the state or on the family. Elaborating the point, she argues that their dependency is not intrinsic to their physical or chronological condition; instead they have been 'socially constructed' as dependent because they are arbitrarily ruled out from being party to the bargain or contract which non-dependent individuals are able or obliged to enter into with society. Hence, systems of support and care may vary according to the degree to which the confinements of the disabled are compounded by the social constraints of marginalisation and stigmatisation, or mitigated by the social supports of integration. In societies which do not have formal segregated care systems, the principal structure of kinship provides the basis for caring. She further states that in situations where the society takes on responsibility for providing care, the form of care adopted has tended to be modelled closely on the familial model. The post-war period has seen a consolidation of guiding objectives underlying formal care policies, promoting dependence on the familial model of care.

In her book dealing with the ideologies of caring, Dalley (1988) has focused on dependent people and women who usually care for them. Dalley highlights the ideology—the pattern of beliefs and attitudes which underlie action. In particular, she deals with the competing ideologies upon which alternative social policies for the provision of care for dependent people are based, namely familism and collectivism.

Analysing the meaning of caring, and taking the example at the affective level, Parker and Graham (in Dalley 1998, 8) state that a distinction can be made between 'caring for' and 'caring about'. The first is to do with the tasks of tending another person; the second is to do with the feelings for another person. Caring for and caring about are deemed to form a unitary, integral part of a woman's nature (which cannot be offloaded in the 'normal' state of affairs). In the 'extra-normal' situation of a child being chronically dependent beyond the constraints of dependency dictated by its age—through sickness and handicap—the mother automatically extends and is expected to extend her 'caring for' function. Just as the affective links which form at birth are tied into the mechanical links of servicing and maintenance in the case of healthy children, the same affective links in the case of disabled and chronically dependent family members get tied to the servicing and maintenance functions.

In the public sphere, the same forces are at work; women go into the caring occupations because their natures and intertwined capacities for caring for and caring about are thought to suit them well for those types of jobs.

The mixing of the caring functions (for and about) has implications for both parties in the caring relationship. Love, in this context, often becomes fractured or distorted by feelings of obligation, burden and frustration. However, the prevailing ethos of family-based care suggests that 'normal' tasks are being performed and roles enacted are straightforward, expected and unproblematic. According to Dalley, evidence suggests that the boundaries of obligation and willingness are indeed carefully delimited and the willingness to care is highly relationship and context specific. As long as a daughter or son with disability is a child, caring falls within the normal parameters (even though it may be arduous). Once the child becomes an adult, tensions in the caring relationship may develop—love, obligation, guilt and dislike may all be intermingled (Dalley 1988).

The ambivalence frequently felt by those involved in the process of caring is made more problematic because public discourse insists that there can be no separation between caring for and caring about. Official and lay commentaries on community care policies all assert the conjunction of the two.

For men, the entanglement of caring for and caring about does not, broadly speaking, exist and where it does, these men are usually regarded as atypical in contrast to women, for whom to disentangle from the process is to be unnatural. Men, it is recognised, can care about, without being expected to care for. A man is expected to provide the setting within which the provision of care may take place and the finances for it, if he has no wife.

Thus, in a society where standards of success are measured in terms of the public sphere of male achievement and where female work, at both home and outside, tends to be dominated by routine, often physically onerous and unrewarding activity, the cost women pay is high. Why do women accept this cost? The common view is that it is located in women's special relationship to the function of caring, their capacities for self-sacrifice and sense of altruism. Both men and women hold this view. This raises the issue of ideology and internalising the values. A view that holds women to be caring to the point of self-sacrifice is propagated at all levels of thought and action; it figures in art and literature, it is present in the social welfare policies and it is the currency in which the social exchanges within the domestic sphere are transacted. Once this central tenet—of women's natural propensity to care (in contradistinction to men's nature)—is accepted, the locus for that caring then becomes determined. With woman as carer, man becomes provider, the foundation of the nuclear family is laid. It becomes the ideal model to which all should approximate.

For most women, especially the working-class women, the model results in the triple burden—child rearing, housework and wage labour. The nuclear family and the roles associated with it may not always exist in concrete form; however, as an ideological construct, it is of crucial significance. Land and Rose (in Dalley 1988, 17) have discussed how the notion of altruism is fundamental to the ways of seeing women in modern society. They call the personal servicing that women do caring for and caring about as compulsory altruism—which encapsulates both the self-sacrifice and selflessness involved and the prescriptive expectations of society that women shall perform that role. Land and Rose show how social policies have been built on the same assumptions to such an extent that the altruism which women come to see as naturally part of their character becomes compulsory. The policies could not be implemented and the structure would not function if women declined to be altruistic. They cite both the Beveridge proposals and current community care policies as examples, suggesting that they reinforce the traditional pattern of enforced dependency and compulsory altruism. This is not to be against the

> Expression of free altruism which potentially lies within community care and self help strategies... the feminist hostility to community care turns partly on the needs and interests of women which are to be masked once more in altruistic services to others and partly on the needs and interests of the cared for. (Dalley 1988, 18)

This, according to Dalley, is the nub of the problem. To be critical of community care policies is not to be critical of the importance of caring for and caring about, or of the necessity of enabling disabled and chronically dependent people to live 'normalised' and 'ordinary' lives. Nor is it to deny that people want to be cared for in familiar surroundings, and to be cared about by people about whom they themselves also care. But because there is consensus at the level of public discourse (both official and lay) that community care is the right policy on both ethical and pragmatic grounds, feminists run the risk of being severely criticised as self-interested and uncaring. It is important that they contest these judgements: To fight for women's rights is to fight for justice just as it is to fight for the rights of any disenfranchised, subordinated or devalued group, and to question the nature of community care is to seek solutions which are equitable, comfortable and acceptable for chronically dependent people as well as for women as (potential) carers.

For the moment, there is widespread acceptance of the way things are. Women have internalised the altruistic ideal; society has capitalised on it. Scathingly, Dalley argues that with women being prepared to remain at or return to the home to care, society is provided with a ready-made 'reserve army' of nurses—an army which does not need hospitals to be built for it to work in and does not need wages to be paid to it, because it is assumed that its members are already provided for by being dependent on and supported by wage-earning men. It is this 'reserve army' which is increasingly being activated to provide the community care that policies and politicians have been calling for over recent years—a form of care that is largely uncosted and unmeasured, which can be invoked by planners and politicians without its costs being borne by official resources. Women are offered little option as to whether they participate as carers or not. Indeed choice is also as well not available to those in need of care.

In a review article published in the *New York Times*, Martha Nussbaum (2001) further develops the arguments on disability and society on the basis of three books on the issue of caring for dependent persons (Berube 1998; Kittay 1998; Williams 1999).

According to Nussbaum, in *Love's Labour*, which is an account of Sesha, a child with disability, Kittay argues that Sesha's need for care suggests both major criticisms of the dominant theories of social justice and major changes that should be made in the political arrangements. To begin with, she poses the question: Who does all the work that extreme dependency requires? In most cases, according to Eva Kittay and Joan Williams, this work is done by women, since women are far more likely than men to accept part-time work and the career detours it requires. Even fathers who agree to help care for a child, who will soon go off to school, moreover are much less likely to shoulder the taxing long-term burden of care for a child or parent with extreme disability. Citing the example of the US, most women who do such work cannot count on much by way of support from an extended family or community network.

Much of the work of caring for a dependent is unpaid; it is not recognised by the market as work. And yet it has a large effect on the life of such a worker, for persons who can afford hired help will find that such work is mostly done by women, who are themselves, even though paid, neither paid highly nor as generally respected by society as they should be for performing a vital social service.

Kittay and Williams posit that a just society may be one that would also look at the other side of the problem, the burdens on people who provide care for dependants. These people may need many things: recognition that what they are doing is work; assistance, both human and financial; and a chance at a rewarding career for themselves and participation in social and political life. Joan Williams shows that it was assumed that women, who were not full citizens anyway and did not need to work outside the home, would do all this work. Women were not asked whether they would do this work, it was just theirs to do.

One now thinks of women as equal citizens who are entitled to pursue the full range of occupations. Also, we now generally think that they are entitled to a real choice about whether they will assume the burden of caring for the extremely dependent. But the realities of life in a society that still assumes that this work will be done for free, 'out of love', continue to put enormous burdens on women across the entire economic spectrum, diminishing their productivity and contribution to civic and political life.

Answering the question on what theories of justice have said about these problems, Nussbaum says that Kittay insists that it is virtually nothing. In fact, Kittay believes that these theories have done real harm, by shaping a person's practical political ideas through their subtle effect on the ways one speaks and thinks. For example, she plausibly suggests that attacks on providing welfare for non-working mothers are influenced by images of the citizen as an independent worker that come to us from centuries of social-contract thinking. Thus, Kittay holds that more perceptive philosophical theorising is important to address these issues in the context or practical political life. Even if not immediately, theoretical conceptions shape public arguments, giving people the concepts they use and shaping the alternatives they consider.

According to Nussbaum, Kittay also suggests that political discourse is pervasively shaped by the idea of society based on a contract for mutual advantage, an idea that has dominated political theory in the Western tradition. All social contract theories adopt a fictional hypothesis that appears innocent: the fiction of competent adulthood. The parties to the social contract are assumed, as John Locke wrote, to be 'free, equal and independent' (in Nussbaum 2001, 35). Contemporary advocates of the social contract theory explicitly adopt such a hypothesis. For instance, the American philosopher David Gauthier stated that people of unusual need are 'not party to the moral relationships grounded by a contractarian theory' (in Nussbaum 2001, 35). Similarly, the citizens in John Rawls' well-ordered society are 'fully co-operating members of society over a complete life' (cited in Nussbaum 2001, 35). Since the partnership envisaged is for the mutual advantage of the contracting parties, provision for people who are not part of the bargain will be an afterthought—not part of the basic institutional structure to which they agree. As Kittay shows, Rawls explicitly omits from the situation of basic political choice the more extreme forms of need and dependency that human beings may experience. Although caring for people who are not independent is a 'pressing practical question', Rawls argues that it may reasonably be postponed to a later legislative stage, after basic political institutions are designed.

Care for children, the elderly and the disabled is a major part of the work that needs to be done in any society, and in most societies it is a source of unfairness. Any theory of justice needs to think about the problem from the beginning, in the design of the basic institutions. Rawls' list of primary goods includes liberties and opportunities, income and wealth, and the social bases of self-respect by which Rawls means the institutional structure ensuring all citizens are treated as having worth and dignity. But care during lengthy periods (or a life) of extreme dependency is never mentioned. According to Nussbaum, Rawls measures relative social position with reference to income and wealth alone, ignoring the possibility that a group denied dignity may not, as a class, be the most deprived economically. Some people with disability are economically disadvantaged and others not. However, all encounter special problems in achieving self-respect that a just society ought to address.

Amartya Sen (in Nussbaum 2001, 36) has criticised Rawls' theory of primary goods: that it ignores the fact that people have varying capacities to convert income and wealth into the ability to function effectively.

Kittay doubts that a liberal theory of justice can adequately address these problems. She feels that Western political theory must be radically reconfigured to put the fact of dependency at its heart. The facts, according to her, are that we are all 'some mother's child' and that we exist in intertwined relations of dependency and this should be the guiding image for political thought. Such a care-based theory, she thinks, is likely to be very different from any liberal theory, since the liberal tradition is deeply committed to goals of independence and liberty. According to Nussbaum, Kittay seems to believe that a care-based theory would support a type of politics that provides comprehensive support for needs throughout all citizens' lives, as in some familiar ideals of the welfare state, but this would be a welfare state in which liberty is far less important than security and well-being. However, Nussbaum points out the inconsistency in Kittay's argument with the example of Kittay's controversial proposal of a direct non-means tested payment to those who care for family dependants at home. This clearly has, or could have, a liberal rationale: that of ensuring that these people are seen as active, dignified workers rather than as passive non-contributors. Further, to be sure, nobody is ever self-sufficient; the independence we enjoy is always both temporary and partial. As Kittay rightly points out, independence should not be seen as a necessary condition of dignity for all people with mental disability, and Nussbaum states that it is good to be reminded of that fact by a theory that also stresses the importance of care of dependent people. But, Nussbaum argues: Is being 'some mother's child' a sufficient image for the citizen in a just society? She thinks we need a lot more: liberty and opportunity and the chance to learn and imagine on one's own. These goals are as important for the disabled as they are for others, though they are much more difficult to achieve.

Michael Berube, discussing the different images of disability, talks of the 'social construction' of various human categories. He writes that both the limitations and the value of that idea became clearer to him as a result of his life with son Jamie. Part of Jamie's condition is clearly not socially created, and Berube gives a detailed genetic and medical account of Down syndrome. But much of Jamie's condition is social: Will he be called a 'Mongoloid idiot'? A 'retarded child'? Or will he get a chance to meet other children as simply 'Jamie', a kid who is a little different, but then children are all different anyway—he is just a little more so? According to Berube, such changes in labelling make a difference. Beyond good attitudes, we need good laws. But both Berube and Kittay are worried about this aspect, for the laws protecting the disability are fragile. They can be easily undone, particularly in a society determined to decrease the public sector. Berube's anxiety is about the current view that people, who are not 'productive' in a narrow economic sense, are a drag on the whole society.

This takes one to the issue of the caregivers. Both Williams and Kittay see the work of caring for dependants at home as a crucial issue, affecting the social equality of women. They hold the view that women are often subtly coerced by social norms into shouldering the burden of caring for a dependent. Williams argues that any solution to the problem has different parts—one is the reallocation of domestic responsibilities between men and women in the home. The second is the role of the state. The state may lighten the burden of people who care for the dependants through a wide range of policies.

Ending the review, Nussbaum considers Berube right in suggesting that the key to social justice for both the disabled and those who care for them lies in enlarging the imagination. If fellow citizens are not seen as parties to a mutually advantageous bargain, then one will never see value in the permanently handicapped. Value in the disabled elderly is seen only in terms of them as formerly productive people who deserve some recompense for that earlier productivity; this is surely not all that their dignity requires. Another point is that if little value or dignity is seen in dependent people, we will be unlikely to see dignity in the work done dressing or washing them, and we will be unlikely to accord this work the social recognition it should have.

According to Nussbaum, although in both theory and practice American society has moved beyond earlier versions of the social contract tradition, by insisting on human dignity as a central social value, it is far from having shaken off a dark implication inherent in the very idea of a social bargain for mutual advantage, namely that those who remain dependent are not full participants. Thus, Gauthier says that while the elderly have paid for the care they receive by earlier periods of productivity, the disabled have not. Berube's phrase that 'a more capacious and supple sense of what it is to be human' is crucial according to Nussbaum if we, as a society, are to think more clearly about problems of justice (Nussbaum 2001).

SOCIAL SUFFERING

It is said that humankind's most fundamental beliefs are those that concern life, suffering and death. This leads to efforts to prolong life, alleviate suffering and prevent death, bringing into focus specifically the roles of the medical sciences and health care strategies and generally the social, economic and political contexts of their development.

Social suffering brings into a single space an assemblage of human problems that have their origins and consequences in the devastating injuries that social forces can inflict on human experience (Kleinman et al. 1997, ix). Social suffering results from what political, economic and institutional power does to people and reciprocally from how these forms of power themselves influence responses to social problems. Included under the category of social suffering are conditions that are usually divided among separate fields, conditions that simultaneously involve health, welfare, legal, moral and religious issues. They destabilise established categories. For example, the trauma, pain and disorder to which atrocity gives rise are health conditions; yet they are also political and cultural matters. Similarly, poverty is the major risk factor for all ill health and death; yet this is only another way of saying that health is a social indicator, and indeed a social process. The clustering of various problems or disorders such as substance abuse, street violence, domestic violence, AIDS and tuberculosis among people runs against the professional medical idea that sufferers experience one or at most two major problems at a time. That grouping of human problems also defeats categorisation of such issues, principally psychological or medical and therefore individual. Instead, it points to the often-close link of personal problems with societal problems. It also reveals the interpersonal grounds of suffering; in other words, it reveals that suffering is a social experience. Social suffering is shared across high-income and low-income societies, primarily affecting in such settings those who are desperately poor and powerless. Although the subject of suffering cannot be examined as a single theme or a uniform experience, it is profoundly social, and the instances giving rise to it are not merely a correlation but a causal web in the global political economy (Kleinman 1995).

According to Kleinman, suffering as a social experience, in the Western tradition, lays emphasis on the subjective feelings of the afflicted individual, which is often viewed as isolated and forlorn. This is the dominant analytic paradigm for understanding suffering that results from serious chronic illness and disability. Framed this way, suffering becomes the pain, hurt, loss and search for meaning of a unique person who alone must bear the deep burden of his/ her troubles. Thus, the paradigmatic locus of suffering is the private space of the person with the problem. However, from the study of the Chinese society in particular, Kleinman has argued that the locus of suffering should be in the inter-subjective space of interactions, especially families. Viewed this way, suffering is a mode of social experience. The point is not to minimise the seriousness of problems faced by the individual patients but rather to appreciate the importance that they and their families attribute to the interpersonal, relational locus of hardship among the family members. This inter-subjective sensibility frequently leads family members to emphasise their own adversity as equivalent to or even greater than the patients' experience.

The focus of concern is on the family and its members. What is most at stake in suffering is the abridgement of the family's aspiration, the threat to the family's life chances, and the loss and hurt of the others. The family's success is as much the means of fulfilment of its individual members. The self is its roles and relations with others in the family (and, in turn, with their collective and individual network). Therefore, suffering is as much the inter-subjective experience of parents, spouses, siblings and children as that of the sick person.

Appreciating the implications of the inter-subjective experience of suffering may begin with understanding its epistemological and moral basis, but it eventually requires that we understand suffering as a different way of living illness in the social world. Even within the family, the social experience of suffering is not homogeneous and it may even be divided. Some may even attempt to escape from it. Often mothers and wives cannot refuse but must endure. Epilepsy or any other chronic illness or disability may create a family 'tragedy', whose burden is different for different family members.

Concluding their study, Kleinman et al. (1995) state that the biomedical idea naturalises the illness experience as based solely on pathology. The social course of epilepsy indicates that epilepsy develops in a local context where economic, moral and social institutional factors powerfully affect the lived experience of seizures, treatment and their social consequences. The social course of epilepsy is, therefore, plural, heterogeneous and changing.

Kleinman et al. further state that the central issues for public health policy have been to provide access to health services that can deliver effective treatment and to focus on preventive causes. Framing epilepsy in terms of its social course suggests that to improve the quality of life and reduce disability, it is essential that health and social policy address the local context of social experience. Stigma, institutional discrimination, the relatively high cost of care in a setting of chronic deprivation and the social resistance borne by sufferers are as important for health and health policy as are basic medical services. They are as salient for the content of medical care as are diagnosis and pharmacology. Thus, Arthur Kleinman argues that the social course of illness constitutes much of what is meant by prognosis.

To sum up, Kleinman et al. argue,

> Epilepsy in China as elsewhere indicates that health policy is inseparable from social policy and that social policy is inseparable from social theory. Especially salient is the powerful constraint of circumstances of deep deprivation, which affect so many globally. In order to join social and health policy, narratives as well as numbers, social services along with health services and social theory together with health science perspectives, must have a place in policy formulation. (Kleinman et al. 1995)

CONCLUSION

An attempt has been made in this review of the literature on disability that has facilitated the conceptualisation of the experience of disability which is at the heart of this work. It is important to reiterate that suffering is not really a matter of individual experience and choices but is determined by the larger social, political and economic contexts within which individuals lead their lives. The various case studies cited here have dealt with different regions, categories of people and settings, and all reveal facets of a similar reality, especially for the marginalised. As Paul Farmer says, 'The capacity to suffer is clearly part of being human. But not all suffering is equal' (in Kleinman et al. 1997, 272) in spite of suggestions to the contrary. It is possible to speak of extreme human suffering and recognise at the same time that those living in poverty currently endure an inordinate share of this sort of pain. It is the marginalised of today's world: women, the poor and other discriminated categories who are the chief victims of structural violence—a violence that has escaped the analysis of many seeking to understand the nature and distribution of extreme suffering. We need to recognise that 'it is the poor who are not only more likely to suffer but also that they are more likely to have their suffering silenced' (Paul Farmer, cited in Kleinman et al. 1997, 272). Some of the features of suffering, discussed here, will help us to understand the experiences of the disabled and their families.

PART 2

Making Sense of the Narratives I

Experiencing Disability—
Inter-class Dimensions

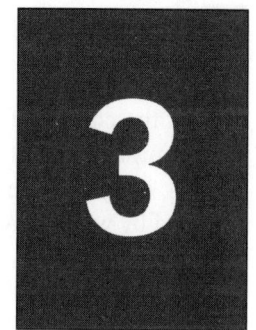

THE ACT OF DIAGNOSIS AND INITIAL REACTION

The narratives I collected as part of my data based on interviews with persons with disabilities and/or their families reveal certain patterns, and a number of points emerge for discussion. To begin with, it is apparent that left to their own devices in a hostile social environment, parents have had to find their own mechanisms of handling their child's disability. The accounts of almost all parents point to the very basic nature of medical knowledge prevalent about CP 20 or more years ago. This meant that the parents did not really get to know what was wrong with their child's development.

Additionally, the manner in which information about the nature of the disability was handled by the medical profession at that time left a great deal unstated. In the absence of precise medical information, the parents could only attribute the disability to the 'lack of oxygen at the time of the birth of the child', or to 'a fever suffered during infancy'. At no point did the medical profession reveal to the parents what the 'specific' condition of the child was, or what the future would entail for the child concerned or for the parents. The routine 'solution' offered by the professional was to ensure that 'exercises' were done regularly so that the child would become capable of some level of independence. The birth of a child with a disability thus remained a situation beyond the control of the parents, something for which the parents were completely unprepared. On the basis of accounts provided by parents, Ghai writes eloquently about the emotions that parents are engulfed by when they 'discover' that their child is disabled:

> The ordeal begins with the very act of diagnosis. Doctors and allied professionals tend to avoid breaking the news, typically offering a cause for disability after the child's birth, giving the news abruptly or failing to give the parents the true picture of the disability. Presumably this is done to reduce the stress of the situation, although each measure may serve only to increase parental feelings of futility and hopelessness. (Ghai 2010)

The way the doctor handles the task of giving the information is very important in determining the course of action that the parents are going to take. For instance, in the case of Gulbano (Gulbano, interview with the author, Chennai, 2011), who has two children with CP, the doctors did not tell her or the family that the child has a disability in either of the cases. In both cases, they were told that the baby has a problem but did not specify the nature of the problem or how to deal with it. The only information they were given was to take the baby to a physiotherapist.

In the case of Shankaran, there seems to have been an apparent emergency situation of the baby having an oxygen deficit, which increased the likelihood that the child could have a disability, but the doctors do not seem to have acted responsibly in providing information, except stating something about delayed milestones.

While in Shankaran's case the doctors at least told the mother (Shankaran's mother, interview with the author, Chennai, 2011) that there would be delayed milestones, in Rekha's case, there was no such information given. According to Rekha's mother (Rekha's mother, interview with the author, Chennai, 2011), the baby was a full-term baby but because of lack of oxygen at the time of delivery, the mother had to have emergency C-section, but the doctors never told the family that something would be wrong. However, the mother says that by the time the baby was three months old, she knew that there was some problem because she had no neck control.

Even in the case of Prakash (Prakash's mother, interview with the author, Chennai, 2011), where it was fairly obvious that there could be a problem due to prolonged labour and the umbilical cord around the baby's neck, the mother was unaware of her child's condition until the child was about seven–eight months old.

In Arun's case (Arun's mother, interview with the author, Delhi, 2005), the mother discovered that her child was not like other children only at the age of two years, since the child was not sitting or crawling.

In some cases, the parents were fortunate that they were at least told the cause of the condition. For instance, in the case of Ashok (Ashok's mother, interview with the author, Delhi, 2005), who was born at home but had no birth cry, he was rushed to Rohtak Medical Hospital. On the second or third day, when the father went to the hospital, the doctor frankly told him that the child would be disabled for life, though mentally he would be alert but physically 'he would not be able to do anything'.

Similarly, Akbar (Akbar's mother, interview with the author, Delhi, 2005), who was a breech baby born at home but had no birth cry, too was rushed to a government hospital and kept in an incubator for almost 15 days. The mother recounts the ordeal of the hospital visits for his *dimaag ka ilaaj* (treatment of his brain).

At least in these cases the parents were given some information that the child would have delayed milestones. However, there are also cases in which the parents are not told anything. For instance, Chanda's mother narrates her experience of the government hospital doctor's response in terms of not telling the parents anything about the diagnosis and condition. The doctor only told them to take her back to the village and feed her *khichdi* (mix of rice and lentils) and banana.

In another instance, Shyama (Shyama, interview with the author, Delhi, 2001) took her older son Sonu to the doctor when he was about six-seven months old, since she realised that the baby was not responding to things, was not making sounds, was not smiling, and was not recognising even her. When the doctor saw him, he told the parents to just play music for him and then he would be fine. The mother was disgusted with the doctor's response because there were other problems such as his stunted growth, low weight and frequent episodes of fits, apart from the lack of social responses that had not been attended to.

Educated parents too were often at a loss to understand the reasons why their child was ill or different from other children, and what had caused the condition of disability.

According to Neerja (Neerja, interview with the author, Delhi, 2011), her son, Guddu, had a strange fever roughly every weekend for a few months, which seemed to have affected his motor skills. As the doctors in Delhi were unable to diagnose the condition, on the advice of family and friends the parents took him to England for a medical opinion. However, doctors even there were not able to precisely diagnose the condition and they decided to return to India. Unable to understand what the child's condition was going to be over the years, Neerja heard about two little urchin boys in a village near Delhi who could make predictions and provide some kind of diagnosis. She spent almost the whole day waiting for her turn to come. Then, finally, they made Guddu lie down on the ground and just simply said in Hindi '*dimaag ka lakhwa*', the equivalent of CP. Until then, she had not heard any doctor mention CP. It was only on one of the trips to the hospital about six months after this incident that she heard some doctor mention CP. It was then that she thought, 'My God, those 7 year olds had told me exactly this and it has taken the medical profession such a long time to diagnose Guddu'.

Even parents having a child in the US have been faced with diagnosis and communication difficulties. Arun Shourie and his wife were in Washington when they were expecting their first child. Suddenly, the pregnancy became complicated; there was a premature delivery and the baby was put into an incubator. Following injections and blood transfusions, the parents discovered in a roundabout way that something had gone wrong as there had been, over a point of time, insufficient oxygen in the incubator. The baby was in the incubator for a month. Three months later, the parents were told that the baby's brain had suffered an injury and he had CP, which was then a new word—a word that was being used to 'raise a lot of money' as the doctor put it. However, at that time, even in the US it meant nothing except that parents would be told how their child was faring against the milestones. But again, as the doctor said, that was something the parents would notice themselves anyway (Shourie 2011).

The attitude of the medical profession over the years despite greater awareness about disability and medical advancements does not seem to have undergone much change. Parents are still unaware of why their children are not going to be like others and what lies in store for them as a family in the future.

Apart from the misinformation or lack of diagnosis, the medical profession is also insensitive in the way it handles children with disability. For instance, it is not unusual, even now, for a doctor to refuse to help out a child who may have something as simple as a cold, because it is feared that something 'will go wrong'. It is almost as if a child with disability is subject to a different medical pattern than a 'normal' child is. In the case of Gudiya (Gudiya's parents, interview with the author, Delhi, 2001), the senior doctors of a government hospital refused to handle the case when she broke her jaw, dismissing it as too risky. It was only because of the courage of a junior doctor, who went against the orders of his senior and performed the requisite surgery under local anaesthesia, that Gudiya's ability to eat, speak and give that lovely smile, which is so characteristic of her, was restored.

Another instance is that of Mohan's mother (Mohan's mother, interview with the author, Delhi, 2001), who said that there should be doctors who would be willing to diagnose and give medicines to children with CP whenever they have minor colds or sore throat. Most of the doctors the parents encountered, especially in private clinics or nursing homes, refused to help out or were scared of handling such a case. They would then have to travel to one of the bigger government hospitals even for routine treatment.

At whatever stage information that the child is going to be disabled is actually provided, it triggers a number of questions in the minds of the parents. The most common reaction is the question: 'Why me?' Or 'Why us?' Or 'Why him/her?' (i.e., the child). However, this question does not necessarily come immediately; it is a question which comes up when the intensity of the situation deepens and the parents start living with the situation and facing the challenges that come with it. The most common initial reaction is that of shock followed by grief. For instance, Akbar's mother described her initial reaction to the news that her child would be disabled and, therefore, stigmatised. Her reaction was that he has been born out of her womb so what can people say? He is her child no matter how severely disabled he may be, at least he is not blind and deaf also. Thus, she took solace in the fact that he did not have multiple disabilities.

Mohsin's mother's (Mohsin's mother, interview with the author, Delhi, 2005) initial reaction was of being very upset when she got to know about his condition. And he was the first born too. But they stated that with a heavy heart they have accepted him, and he is their child so they have to look after him.

Arun's mother recounted her initial reaction quite graphically: When she heard about her son's condition, she was very upset. She stopped eating and drinking, going out or interacting with neighbours or even with people who would come over, even relatives. She thought about her son constantly, his condition, how she would manage, what the future holds for him and her and why did she have such a child.

Shakti's mother (Shakti's mother, interview with the author, Chennai, 2011) recounted the shock when they got to know that her child had CP from the doctor who delivered their second child. Her husband was totally shattered on hearing the information and till date has not recovered from the shock. Listening to all the accounts of the kind of life for a person with CP would be, the mother fainted.

ACCESS TO SERVICES

From a time when there were no significant services available for people with disabilities (about three decades ago) to now when not only services are available but technology too, the issue of access to these facilities still remains very important for parents of children with disabilities. Almost all the narratives, irrespective of the socio-economic class location, indicate that the presence of a child with disability in the family led them to realise that there are 'such types of children too', that is, those with CP. Many of them knew that that there were persons with blindness and deafness and persons with a 'deformed' limb or two or who were mentally slow. Thus, the awareness about services for children with CP was not present in their consciousness. It is very obvious that the more the resources, especially financial resources a family have, the more the services can be accessed. This fact is borne out in the narratives too. For instance, people belonging to the higher economic classes were even able to consult doctors abroad for diagnosis, prognosis, and line of rehabilitation, and were able to get the benefit of early therapeutic services abroad.

The access to services is an issue from the time of birth, especially in rural and slum areas where often the hospital is very far and getting to it in time can often cause precious time to be lost. The distance from the hospital often leads the family to have the baby delivered at home by a dai (auxiliary nurse; midwife). For instance, in the case of Amit, the mother (Amit's mother, interview with the author, Delhi, 2005) had just travelled a long distance by bus to her in-laws' place in Ballabhgarh. The mother narrates the story of Amit's birth thus: They decided to have the delivery of the baby at home instead of in the hospital because the hospital was very far. The journey earlier in the day to the hospital for a check-up had exhausted her a lot, and she was unable to undertake the return journey. It was night by the time the baby was born. He was very thin, underweight and extremely weak, and the doctor who did the delivery then exclaimed that the baby was born before time and that they should have waited. The doctor gave the baby a bath. By the morning the baby turned yellow and had developed jaundice of a very severe nature. Her mother-in-law told her not to worry and that sometimes a weak baby does get jaundice. For three days he had no urinary or bowel movements; this caused some anxiety. Then they decided to take him to the government hospital in Ballabhgarh itself. When they reached the hospital and the doctor started examining him, the baby finally passed urine. So, then they brought him back home. In the next 15 days, there was no improvement in his jaundice condition. Then they took him to Kalawati hospital in Delhi about which they had heard from others. The doctor there examined him and said that he had been brought too late and that his brain had been affected. They admitted him for 15 days to treat the jaundice but could not tell them then exactly how much of his brain had been damaged. After 15 days when the jaundice was cured and they brought him home, they noticed that he could not hold his neck—it would dangle. Even after so many years the mother wonders whether Amit would not have become disabled had the hospital been more accessible.

Another instance of the lack of access to medical facilities exemplifying the crucial and precious loss of time that could have provided more opportunity for critical early intervention is shown in Vibha's case. The mother (Vibha's mother, interview with the author, Delhi, 2005) narrates that she was taken to the local hospital as she developed some pains, but the doctors reassured the family that nothing was the matter and sent her back home. After she reached home, again the next day she felt some discomfort and was taken to a nearby hospital different from the previous one as there was a strike in the government hospitals. The doctor was called, and she said there was nothing to worry and that there is still a lot of time for the baby to come. However, the mother felt that the baby might be born any moment as she already had the experience of giving birth to a baby (Vibha's brother). By the night, the situation seemed to have gotten worse because the doctors advised the family to take her immediately to AIIMS in Delhi. The family rushed and arranged a vehicle to go to Delhi, but they had barely reached the Delhi border when her condition started deteriorating in terms of excruciating pains. She was admitted to the closest hospital on the way and had the baby. As soon as the baby was born, her husband took the baby to AIIMS in a hired vehicle and admitted the baby to the ICU.

In the case of Mohsin, the family had to go from one hospital to another seeking medical attention on the day of the birth. The mother recounts the ordeal of having the baby in a private nursing home. He was born through a normal delivery and he had a normal birth cry. But soon after he was delivered, he had severe hiccups. They were told by the doctors to take him to a bigger hospital. They took him to Pant government hospital, where he was supposed to be put on oxygen. But it was not available. The Pant hospital doctor told them to take him to Kalawati children's hospital. So, a lot of time was lost in going from one hospital to the next. At Kalawati they put him on oxygen. He recovered a little and the doctors told them to take him home. After they brought him home he started getting fits. So, they took him back again to Pant hospital instead of Kalawati hospital. There the doctor explained to them that because of the delay in getting oxygen, his brain had been affected and he would not be like a normal child.

Further, when Mohsin used to be taken to the hospital for the treatment of his seizures, the ordeal was too much for them as there used to be a long line at the hospital, and waiting used to be quite traumatic. Holding Mohsin in the lap was difficult. The mother narrates how she used to make him lie on the floor of the hospital on a bed sheet. And if he got a fit during the wait, it used to be very difficult to manage, the doctor or nurse would not even come and attend to him or hurry up the process for him. They used to give the medicine only for about 15 days to a month and insisted that each time the child should be brought to the hospital for more medicine.

This situation forced them to go to a private clinic in Meerut. According to the mother, the conditions were easier there since they did not have to take Mohsin every time and anyone could go and get the medicine.

Rumi's (Rumi's mother, interview by the author, Delhi, 2005) example could even be considered a case of medical negligence since the ultrasound report prior to the birth showed that the baby was in a breech position, and C-section should have been done. But there was no doctor available at night when they went to the hospital for the delivery of the baby. She told the nurse that her labour pains seem to have started and requested to call the doctor. The nurse just asked her to turn on her side and go to sleep. The mother questioned her suggestion since she already had experienced giving birth to two children; so, she knew that it was labour pains and not just discomfort. And very shortly after this conversation her labour pains increased, but there was no doctor around. She had had an ultrasound earlier and all the regular tests did not reveal anything except that the baby was in a breech position. She was supposed to have an operation in the evening around 7 PM, but they did not do it. She did not know the reason for the delay and by 6 AM the baby was born. If only they had done the operation on time, this condition may not have been there.

It is important to note that there is a skewed network of services available for the persons with disability. Despite being a signatory to international declarations, the government is still working in the framework of the medical model and limiting its role to only providing prosthetics. In the absence of a state network of access and supportive facilities for persons with disabilities, the NGO sector has taken up some of the responsibility. Unfortunately, the NGOs are located primarily in the urban centres, and even within the urban centres in localities which have middle to upper class families. In this situation, it is not only the rural areas but even slum areas which remain neglected and have no access to NGO services.

Although the situation is changing slightly now with some NGOs having an outreach programme in the slums and rural areas, the facilities are mainly limited to basic assessments and distribution of aids and appliances. Thus, children with disabilities particularly are left out of the schooling system, vocational training and employment opportunities. Those who are able to benefit from some of the schemes are mainly those who are able to move around and express themselves to some extent to access the various schemes.

For instance, in Mohsin's case, he gets severe and multiple fits (almost 8–10 fits a day). To get treatment for the fits, the parents used to take him to the local government hospital. The mother describes her struggle of going to the government hospital and how it used to be almost a day-long engagement. They would have to go early in the morning: Getting both kids ready was quite tough, especially in winter. Then the father would have to take the day off. In addition, it used to be quite expensive because they would have to hire an auto-rickshaw that used to charge ₹150 one-way.

In the case of Jagan (Jagan's mother, interview with the author, Chennai, 2011), who got seizures following a fever when he was about three and a half years old, the mother recounts how the seizures kept coming continuously for three months they were in the hospital. After returning from the hospital, they still had to take him daily to the hospital for check-up. Staying at the hospital was not only expensive but also difficult because they had to look after the other children left at home. The doctors at the hospital told them that some permanent damage had happened to the brain and the chances of recovery were very remote. Every day for three years he was taken to the hospital. While the medical expenses were not too much because it was a government hospital, however, the daily commuting even by bus was quite a lot at the time. Because they spent the whole day at the hospital, they also had to purchase some food for tiffin. Therefore, additional costs were quite high.

In the case of Tejas (Tejas' mother, interview with the author, Delhi, 2005) in rural Haryana, by the time there was access to services, or rather by the time an NGO reached his village with some services, he was already about 17–18 years old, his spasticity had increased and he was unable to sit on the wheelchair given to him free of cost in some medical camp; as a result, he has remained bed-ridden from birth.

On the other hand, when Malini's parents could not find anything in India by way of services to cater for their daughter's needs, the family relocated to England in order to access services that would improve their daughter's life. This was possible because a variety of financial as well as social network resources worked in their favour (Chib 2011a).

TRANSPORT

Access to services is severely hampered across classes due to a small but very significant reason, which is that of transport. While families that are better off financially are able to make multiple rounds to doctors and therapists because of their private transport, the situation for those without private transport highlights the dismal state of public transport in our country. This further adds to the inaccessibility of services whether provided by the government or an NGO. Gulbano, who belongs to a lower income group, narrated that despite living in the capital city there was no economical private transport available, and they also needed to pay for the therapy sessions. She had to use the public transport to take her two sons with CP for their daily exercise therapy. Since her husband could not accompany her every day and she could not carry both the children while travelling, the following was her routine: Before taking her elder son for his session, she prepared food for the younger one, fed and put him to sleep and locked him up. Then she carried her elder son in the bus for his therapy. It used to take half an hour to reach. After his session was over, she carried him back, fed him, and put him to sleep and then took the younger one for his session; again travelling to and fro by bus. And the whole day went like that.

Ashok's mother talks not only about the lack of transportation but also about the condition of roads which further prevents access to services. She said that just to take him from home to the petrol pump where the bus came, which was at the end of the road, she had to carry him but was unable to do so because he was a full-grown adult and very heavy. The ordeal of requesting people to help her still haunts her. But if there was a proper road, she could have taken him in the wheelchair and would not have needed to be beholden to anyone. It also meant that he was homebound, and someone always had to be at home to take care of him while the mother went out to do even minor chores. Apart from that, he even got deprived of seeing the world!

Amit's mother recalls taking him to Kalawati hospital in Delhi from her house in rural Haryana. She used to take him every day by herself, carrying him in the train, and then by bus to the hospital from the station to get the exercises done. She used to leave early in the morning and return in the evening. The stress was so much that she herself started getting fits (seizures) during the journey.

In the case of Rekha, who lived outside of Chennai, when the parents discovered there was a problem with the baby they took her to a neurosurgeon, who referred them to a special school in Chennai. Rekha was admitted in the home-based programme of the special school. This required the mother to go every month with Rekha, learn the programme and tasks and follow them at home. The mother narrates how she used to go back to her native place and do that programme for one month and then again come back to Chennai with Rekha. But this constant coming and going every month became very difficult and was very expensive as well.

Even going out for social occasions is tough for the family which does not have the adequate transport or resources. For instance, in Sundar's case (Sundar's parents, interview with the author, Delhi 2001), the family does not travel out of station because of the hassles of taking the wheelchair and the inaccessibility of the toilet.

In contrast to the above instances of difficulty in accessing services to the absence of adequate transport facilities, resources such as private transport make all the difference. Guddu, who lives in the national capital city, could attend a local private primary school up to the age of 14 years. This was made possible not only because the principal of the school was a broad-minded person, but also because the parents could afford a car and driver solely for Guddu. They could also afford a maid exclusively to look after Guddu and be with him at the school throughout the duration he was there.

Guddu, thus, had a community to interact with and a routine in which he used to get ready, go out and then return. Although Guddu cannot communicate verbally, he obviously liked the routine because he did not show any distress about going out or being in the school. The parents finally withdrew him because his health was not very good, and it was difficult for him to get up early in the morning and follow the school routine. Apart from this, the parents were also registered for the home-based programme in which people from the SSNI used to come to the house to help with therapeutic and educational interventions.

PHYSICAL SPACE OF THE HOUSE

Many of the parents in urban areas live in rented accommodation, while in the rural areas they mostly own the house. The physical space of the house is something that is generally overlooked by most builders, so that it is made disabled friendly even though more awareness campaigns are going on today. Most families are not able to use a wheelchair in the house; hence, they have to carry the person with disability from one room to another, from the bed to the toilet or down the stairs to go out as there are no lifts. In many houses, especially in the rural areas and slums, there are no toilets on the premises; either they have to go to the fields in the rural area or go to the public toilet in the slum. The need for such a facility within the house is highlighted through the case of Tejas in rural Haryana. A toilet was built in his house with the help of the NGO and panchayat. This made it easier for the mother to clean up the child as well as accord some dignity to Tejas. In the slums, it is often a pathetic scene to see the person with disability struggle to get to the public toilet. Sometimes parents make some temporary arrangement for the person in the house or just outside the house for the toilet functions. As there is no proper sewage system in the slums and rural areas, it is often difficult to make a toilet in the house.

The rooms in a rented accommodation are also quite small and a wheelchair is often kept in the drawing room which becomes a mere showpiece, rather than being used in the house. This is because there is hardly any space in the house to manoeuvre the wheelchair. Further, it is often difficult to get accommodation of one's choice, such as a ground floor house. In some houses, the rooms are on one floor and the toilet, often a shared one, on another.

In the case of the higher income group, the houses are often their own, spacious enough for a wheelchair to go through the doors. The person with disability has his/her own room with some space for the caregiver to stay in the room itself. The toilet is often modified for the special needs of the child. There is often a small garden into which the person with disability can be wheeled for the winter sun or summer evenings.

NEED FOR SPACE

From the discussion above, it is apparent that apart from just the need for physical space there is a desperate need for social and psychological spaces in which parents as well as the child can express themselves. While parents are now seeking ways by which it becomes possible for the growing child with disability to be in touch with other people, organisations are not adequately prepared to cater for such needs due to the several constraints mentioned earlier. At the same time, the family's social interactions have come to be severely restricted for a number of reasons, like the difficulties of sustaining a social network in the face of a hostile and stigmatising society. In most cases, interaction remains confined to the extended family. In the course of recounting their lives, one rarely come across the parents talking of taking their child to their friends' place or of friends dropping in for an occasional social visit to spend time with the parents. The situation is one of a bind wherein both social and familial relations are amongst the same people: The parents, siblings and the person with disability are a socially isolated island, since the public typically cannot understand the child with disability's situation.

The need for social and psychological space, particularly in the case of the person with disability, is evident in Natarajan's account of a plan for a summer camp that was designed for a group of mild to moderate CP adolescents. When they discovered that their parents wanted to accompany them, they rebelled against the idea—the whole point of the summer camp for them was that they would be away from home and that included their parents! The students went up to Natarajan and told her quite forthrightly that they did not want their parents in the summer camp with them. According to her, the parents were being overprotective and sheltering their children too much, so that the children had no life outside of their parents.

However, another way of looking at parental overprotectiveness is that although it may be excessive, the social support network is so negligent that the parents in their attempt to ensure some entertainment for the children have themselves become their primary 'entertainers' since this is not recognised by anyone else as a need. Natarajan highlights the different levels at which the parents have to take responsibility for their child with disability by displaying their active participation in every aspect of the child's life, not just in physical caring.

In the cases of parents belonging to the higher income group, there is a social network of friends of parents and extended family who keep dropping by. As a result, the child with disability gets to interact with them as well as their children. The presence of a social network also helps the child in the growing years to befriend not only peers but also adults who may become close confidants of the person with disability. For instance, both Malini and Soni have a small but relatively close circle of friends with whom they can develop their own relationships. In the case of Samina, the hostel at the organisation provided that opportunity to befriend young professionals and others. Even for persons such as Adit (Shourie 2011) and Guddu, who may not be able to interact in a very involved way as Malini or Soni, the social network does provide an opportunity to come out of the island of parents, caregivers and other family members. The social network also helps to make it possible for the family to go out on holidays. The available resources help the family to take the person with disability comfortably on trips in India as well as abroad. This is not the case in many of the families belonging to the lower socio-economic groups.

It is necessary to recognise that the parents too need psychological and social spaces for themselves. This is something they perhaps cannot articulate to the world outside, and maybe not even to themselves, caught up as they are in the stereotype of the *sevabhav* that is expected of them. Thus, Shyama, the mother of two children with disabilities, who has absolutely no time to herself and is worn out with work, has had to be medically advised by her doctor to go out of her house for a while every day as a way of switching off from her duties as a mother, caring for her disabled sons. The need for social and psychological space is also articulated by Shyama who talks of the need for 'space' more in physical terms, expressed in the desire to go back to the village, a more open space where life would be 'easier'.

However, the revelations of the study of 41 villages of Andhra Pradesh indicate that the need for 'space' is very much a psychological one, emanating from a feeling of being trapped in a situation rather than merely in a physical space. The romantic notion of life being easier 'there' is dispelled in the case of a mother with two children with disabilities, one aged three and the other five, who lives in a village: 'The mother wept and said that she had not been able to leave her home even once in the past five years because of the unrelenting need to take care of the children' (Mander 2002, 112).

In the case of the upper income groups, the need for space is met by the resources and the available support of extended family, friends and hired caregivers, to look after the person with disability in the absence of one, or at times both parents. For instance, in the case of Guddu or Malini, the mothers who were both working and required to undertake work-related travel, were able to continue to do so because of the support structure. In one instance, Guddu's mother had taken him for a holiday to the hills, and from there she had to go abroad for a meeting. She was able to do so without upsetting Guddu's holiday because of the support network that she had.

This leads us to examine the issue of whether institutions actually cater, or can cater, for the 'felt needs' of not only an educational and vocational nature but also the emotional and social needs of the persons with disabilities and their parents. Given the meagre facilities that are available to the disabled and their families, it appears that there is a long way to go to meet the felt needs of the disabled.

As a provision for long-term care, especially for the profoundly and severely affected persons with disability, institutions have not been seriously regarded as a support service in the Indian context. As a result, the only types of services provided by institutions are for prevention, detection and early training of the person with disabilities. The Western model of the institution as a 'modern' institution, which can take over the caring function otherwise performed by families, has not been considered. However, the case of Erwadi and the study of 41 villages in Andhra Pradesh (Wadhwa 2001, 52–54) reveal that there is a need for institutional support of a kind, redesigned perhaps as caring support for long-term care needs, especially for the profoundly and severely affected persons with disability. The report on Andhra Pradesh describes how the disabled are left without food and care for long periods as families go out to labour. Erwadi brings out the indigenous variant of the institutional solution to care, linking it to faith and traditional healing beliefs, a system existing outside of the state structure. This leads us to think about locating the issues of the rights of the disabled, and of care and caregiving, in a broader political economy and cultural context. Neither from the narratives of the disabled nor from the secondary writing on disability, do we get a picture of either the state or alternative traditional structures actually providing any significantly feasible, humane and acceptable ways of giving care to those who need it from the viewpoint of the disabled and their families.

STIGMA

A painful feature that emerges very clearly from almost all the narratives, irrespective of the socio-economic class, is the fact that the stigma attached to having a person with disability in the family does not really ever go. For instance, a common incident is one that Sundar's parents faced: Once they were told quite bluntly not to bring Sundar to a relative's wedding. Even though they felt upset, the parents still went to the marriage, without Sundar, out of a sense of obligation and to maintain family relations.

The family may be psychologically 'tough' and may come to accept their child with disability, and there could even be certain situations which the family could prepare itself to deal with; for instance, while renting a house it is expected that the family may be discriminated against for having a child with disability. Sundar's father describes the family's experience: After years of shifting from one rented accommodation to another, the family has finally managed to purchase a house of their own. They were driven to buying their own place because, as stated by the father,

> We had a lot of problems in renting an accommodation with such a child. No one would happily accept our situation. The maximum we could stay in one place was a year. Initially the house would be rented to us on sympathetic grounds or whatever. But, then, we would start facing humiliating remarks and many would not like their children or other family members to interact with our children, or with us. It was a torture all those years living on rent.

However, there are also situations for which the family is never really ready: For instance, the stigma the parents have had to face when they tried to get something as basic as medical attention for a cold their child had. The local doctor's blunt refusal to even see the child, and telling the parents to take the child to the government hospital instead, is something no parent could ever be prepared for. It is as if a child with disability has a different medical pattern than the 'normal' child has. In the case of Gudiya, the senior doctors of a government hospital refused to handle the case when she broke her jaw, dismissing it as too risky.

The social stigma of having a child with disability, that too a girl, is heightened in small towns. For instance, in the case of Neetu (Neetu's mother, interview with the author, Delhi, 2001) the paternal grandfather allowed Neetu to attend the town school only up to class 5. The mother recounts why Neetu was not allowed to study further—Neetu's paternal grandfather was some kind of big shot in a small town, and when Neetu was young her condition did not really matter in his social interactions with people around. However, as she grew up, the grandfather started imposing restrictions on her going out or being taken out. He feared his reputation would be at stake and that people would point their fingers at him and talk about his granddaughter's condition.

Gudiya and her parents encountered another kind of stigma. When Gudiya was of schoolgoing age, her parents put her in the local government primary school. Her parents say that they had realised by then that Gudiya was 'not like other children', and they feared that she would be 'caught out' sooner in a private nursery school than in a government school. They also reasoned that, generally, children are not thrown out from a government school. However, by the time Gudiya reached class 2 or 3, the teachers realised that the child was having problems in 'coping' because she could not keep pace with the other children academically. Further, the teachers could not manage her studies as well as her 'behaviour'. The final decision to take Gudiya out of school arose when there were objections being raised by other parents about Gudiya going to the same school as their 'normal' children. It is as if parents of normal children fear that their children too will become 'disabled' in the presence of children with disabilities.

Another form of stigma faced by the family is one which is experienced by the mother of the child: Not only is the child stigmatised for being disabled, but the mother is also stigmatised for bearing 'such' a child. In these situations, while the parents may learn to handle people's comments about their child with disability, the mother is never able to handle the stigma attached to her for having borne 'such' a child, particularly when the husband himself believes that the mother is the 'cause' of the child's disability. The stigma of having a child with disability increases in the cases when the child is born with a disability. In such cases, the mother does feel overwhelmed by the guilt of having borne a child even if no one explicitly holds her responsible. For instance, the mother-in-law of one mother said that 'We have never held her responsible for having given birth to such children; she did not want to have them, did she?' The mother in her interview separately did raise the issue that she has never been explicitly blamed for bearing such children, but there are times when she does think that it may be because of her.

In this context, Gulbano, a mother of two children with CP, says with much hurt and remorse, 'If I am the cause I am also the one suffering the most. They don't have to keep telling me that I did it. These people can't even feel a decimal of the pain that I go through every day'. Another mother of two boys with CP describes how she feels at her office when colleagues discuss their respective children's development vis-à-vis studies, marriage or a job: She sometimes does feel 'ashamed' and burdened.

Ghai describes the mother of a girl with mental disability recounting to her with horror how her sister-in-law told her that it was her own *shrap*, or curse, that was instrumental in giving the parents such a child. Apart from the unequal power within households, in which the daughter-in-law remains the most vulnerable member, what emerges from these instances is that the sheer cruelty of society, as distinct from the negative and discriminative attitudes towards people with disability has been socialised to uphold.

FEELINGS OF HELPLESSNESS, GRIEF AND ANXIETY

The feeling of helplessness of having a child with disability is evident in the responses I got from parents across socio-economic classes during the interviews. In cases where the CP child may have a severe physical disability but is able to speak, communicate and, very importantly, engage intellectually, the feeling of helplessness is relatively less than that in cases of severe multiple disabilities. For instance, there are the cases of Samina, Soni and Malini belonging to different socio-economic classes who are examples of the typical 'intelligent mind trapped in a disabled body' that a person with CP was described as in the early years of the movement to create awareness about the condition. The feeling of helplessness has been relatively milder for all three because the girls have been able to go ahead and make a life on their own, with the opportune support and interventions made at the right time.

A feature across all the narratives, irrespective of socio-economic class, is the implicit and explicit discussion that comes up around the theme of dealing with the realisation that their child is disabled and then having to come to terms with it. Although the mother, in particular, may be going through a certain cathartic release in the course of her routine looking after of the child, the family does go through some kind of a 'grief cycle' when they first discover that the child is disabled. They go through the grief cycle once again when the child reaches the age of 20 or more years. The parents' age, their own ill health, their anxiety about death, along with the fact that the future of the child has to be made secure, consumes them. The tendency of the parents, when the child is younger, is to deal with the situation by responding to the needs of a dependent helpless person—a stage that is not vastly different from that of the parents of 'normal' children, though it involves a great deal more of care. However, there is a point where the needs of the child with disability become very distinctive. Once this distinction is established, or strikes the parents, they begin experiencing the different stages of the grief cycle.

Grief is a process not easily acknowledged in our society: in particular, the grief associated with experiences other than death. Yet grief is an integral part of most life changes and experiences. Some of the emotional responses to grief are shock, anger, guilt, fear, exhaustion, depression, confusion and bargaining. Rando defines grief as 'the process of psychological, social and somatic reactions to the perceptions of loss' (Rando in Pessagno n.d.). The grief cycle or the different stages of grief identified are denial and isolation, anger, depression, bargaining and acceptance.

The grief cycle begins the very moment the parents get the diagnosis that their child will be disabled for life. The parents are suddenly thrown into a new unexpected world, or rather they discover a new world that forces them to accept the fact that their lives are going to be different from those of others. This realisation shatters their understanding of the 'world of perfect beings and perfect lives', a notion many of us are brought up with. The onset of grief comes with the realisation of difference and the non-attainment of the developmental milestones. For instance, Arun's mother describes how she returned from the doctor after hearing about her son's condition: She had stopped eating and drinking, stopped going out or interacting with neighbours or with people who would come over, even relatives. She was constantly thinking about her son, his condition, how she would manage, what the future held for him and her, and why she had such a child. Lalitha's mother describes how she used to cry inconsolably whenever she saw Lalitha having repeated rounds of fits and seizures, when the realisation dawned that she would be disabled and while thinking of what had happened and how she would deal with it.

Similarly Rekha's mother describes how she was very upset when she got to know that Rekha was disabled. She said, 'I would just cry not understanding what had happened, I would not go out, nor even take her anywhere'. As Naresh's mother (Naresh's mother, interview with the author, Delhi, 2005) also said, 'Initially when we got to know it was very difficult to accept as we had high expectations that he would get all right'. Jagan's mother described her grief thus: People around her would look at her sympathetically and used to ask her why she had to look after a child like this. They used to even suggest that she should abandon it, or not feed it or look after it and it would then just wither away. She did not know how to reply to these people and to such comments or suggestions, and would just cry about the situation. Such comments would often make her feel guilty about having borne such a child. But she was in a dilemma about what to do as she did not want, or feel it was right, to abandon such a helpless child.

Shakti's mother describes the parents' grief, 'It was a shock to us when we got to know that he has CP. My husband was totally shattered on hearing the information and has still not recovered from it'. Poonam Natarajan, a professional as well as a parent, and Director, VS, said, she went through two cycles of grief in quick succession. One was when she discovered that her child was spastic and the second, about two years later, when she realised that the child was also mentally retarded. The latter discovery was a feature that had never occurred to her as a possibility and was not a condition she was familiar with. According to Natarajan, the experience of grief is also exacerbated by the fact that there is not enough information available about various disabilities and, especially, about multiple handicaps. This was because the image of the 'model' CP person portrayed until the 1980s was that of an intelligent mind trapped in a crippled body, and most of the CP persons she had interacted with were of average to very high intelligence. She was also not quite sure whether she had ever really overcome the grief of discovering that her child was disabled; in the initial years, every new discovery such as the realisation that 'the child will not walk or will not go to school', was an extremely painful process, and according to her, it is only very gradually that one learns to come to grips with the implications of disability.

It is fairly obvious from the narratives that all the parents, irrespective of their socio-economic class, went through a grief cycle at the point when they 'discovered' that their child was disabled and would be so for life. For instance, when asked about their immediate reaction to the discovery that their child would be disabled, Sundar's father replied that they were not very depressed initially for they did not realise it would be a 'lifelong condition'. Similarly, Nataraj's mother said that initially it was 'a big shock for us. Then we started doctor shopping hoping that some cure would be available'. Naresh's mother describes that there was still some hope for a cure or that a miracle would happen: 'Once we acknowledged that even medically there is nothing much that can be done, we started working on the issue of giving him the best possible life we can give', she said.

Sundar's father's reaction does indicate an underlying facet of grief: The discovery did mark a sense of loss, at whatever stage the realisation dawned on the parents that the disability was a lifelong condition. However, the early reaction was a kind of cover up, or a putting off of the recognition of the disability, in order to deal with the situation. Another instance of one of the consequences of grief is the example of Gudiya's father, whose psychosomatic ailments and narrative continuously showed the anxiety and the cycles or periods of grief he went through. These cycles occurred while he thought about his daughter's situation as it is at present, and, especially, about what it would be in the future.

For parents, the grief does not really go away as there are many occasions which revive it. For instance, Chanda's mother (Chanda's mother, interview with the author, Delhi, 2005) talks about another girl in the neighbourhood who was born at the same time as her, who is now going to college. With tears in her eyes, the mother said, 'When I see that girl and think of Chanda, of how even she would have been going to college, I feel very sad and helpless, but what can I do?' This realisation further compounds her grief and makes the mother ruminate over the situation and she says, 'We are all very saddened and distressed with the situation. At least we can talk and move and be engaged in other things, but more deeply affected than all of us is Chanda because she cannot express or understand anything and is dependent on others for everything—not only for food and toilet functions but also for a simple thing like turning on her side'.

Similarly, a mother of two children with CP describes the grief she feels at the office when her colleagues discuss their respective children's development vis-à-vis studies, marriage or jobs because she has no 'achievements' of her children to share.

Sanjana's widowed mother (Sanjana's mother, interview with the author, Delhi, 2001) recalls how her grief used to be revived every time she went to SSNI. She just could not sit through the parents' workshops which were held in the SSNI. The moment the parents started to talk about their problems, the mother would have tears in her eyes and would want to walk out from there. She felt completely helpless and underconfident of her capacity to cope with Sanjana's situation.

While the grief of the mother is visibly expressed by her, the father is often not able to express it publicly. For example, in Mohan's case, the mother narrated an instance of how one of her husband's friends felt sorry for him and took him to a Sadhavi who asked her husband to 'name the thing that you want'. Her husband replied, 'I have not come to ask for any material thing, I have only come to ask for strength to deal with my *dukh* (grief)'. The Sadhavi was taken aback and did not know how to react to this request. In contrast, Shyama is very articulate in expressing her feelings and state of mind: During the interview, through tears and smiles she narrated the ups and downs of her life. In the beginning, she used to feel that it was not the life she had dreamt of; she also had doubts about whether they were 'bad people that such misfortunes should befall them' and, therefore, 'God was now testing' them.

The grief for parents does not really ever go away since there are many instances that revive it. Sweety's mother (Sweety's mother, interview by the author, Delhi, 2001) acknowledged that even after many years of living with Sweety's condition, she still goes through periods of depression, not so much about 'why we had such a child', but about 'what will her future be'. She feels sad for the kind of life that Sweety will have to live for the rest of her life. The parents feel that all the support and comfort the SSNI provided in the early years when Sweety was placed there had been withdrawn without the realisation that such children once had a routine, had friends and peers in the school, and going to SSNI was also an outing for them. All this is causing the child such mental agony that it is difficult to cope with it; now she cries, is frustrated, is angry and, above all, feels helpless because of her own condition.

Thus, the experience of grief wears many faces at different times in the life cycle for families. Their lives are challenged by change, turmoil, illness, death and/or loss of hopes and dreams. There are many layers to the experience of grief. It is not something that is momentary, it is 'a process' which is cyclical in nature and emerges several times in a lifetime as there are changes in the life course of the family and the person with the disability. The grief is often masked in defence mechanisms. The new challenges that have to be dealt with also make it difficult and painful for the parents to recognise grief at a conscious level and be able to articulate and realise its presence. Different or alternative forms of therapy may be able to bring out the sublimated grief, but there are few facilities for dealing with the feelings of parents. However, exploring these psychological dimensions is beyond the scope of the present study. More needs to be done in this very important field within studies of disability.

The reason the grief resurfaces at different stages and in different forms is because there is also a constant recalibration of expectations through the life cycle of the family and that of the person with disability. As Mohan's mother describes, 'Once the parents have accepted their situation there is nothing which can hurt them, or weaken their determination to look after the child. When parents themselves are disappointed with what they have, it is then that what others say hurts or affects them'. While both parents go through the grief cycle, there may be different ways in which the two express it and deal with it as suggested earlier. It is also found that often it is the mother who is told to be strong, but how to go about that is invariably missing from the counselling or advice. (*This leads to questions of how you are dealt with as a mother.*) According to alternative therapy programmes, unless the mother is rid of her grief, it is transferred to the child, and as a result the child too is unhappy. One of these alternative programmes with which SSNI experimented was bhajan sessions for the parents. Shyama for instance recalls the bhajans and said that they calmed her and gave her a lot of solace and some kind of inner strength to deal with the situation.

Through these narratives one can only get a sense of the grief that is at the surface. It is not possible to get to the core of the grief and whether it is actually fully reconciled is also difficult to assess. This would require one to explore the realm of the existential more deeply. The narratives also open up issues of whether there is really space to grieve—via a kind of grief channel. The emotional acceptance is more difficult than the physical acceptance of the situation. It is this desire for emotional acceptance and the acknowledgement of grief, and subsequently the releasing of grief, which is a very difficult process and often leads parents towards spirituality. Mohan's mother narrates that both parents over time became spiritual. Both of them have taken Diksha (initiation) to serve their child and any such child whom they come across.

On the other hand, for Neerja a way to reconcile her grief is to consider her son Guddu as Rimpoche—one who is forever smiling and accepting things as they come. According to her, it is Guddu who has taught her to accept whatever comes to her in life. It is this aspect of Guddu that gave her the strength to cope with her young daughter's sudden and tragic death. For Gulbano, her two children with CP are her teachers. 'To be very frank my kids are my driving force. My kids have really taught me so many things which I would not have known had I had a normal kid. They have taught me to face life. They have taught me to cope and handle whatever situation that arises'. For Arun Shourie, Adit is the teacher: He says, 'Adit has taught us lessons upon lessons' (Shourie 2011, 15).

Thus, in the mosaic of shock and sense of helplessness, the world of reality is experienced as a 'journey' which the parents, especially the mothers, undertake. As Neetu's mother says—it is a personal tragedy that the mother is still trying to resolve. The findings within the narratives corroborate what studies as well as the field experience of professionals have drawn attention to, that is, families with a disabled member do go through what is called the grief cycle. For example, both Renu Singh and Anuradha Naidu talked about the fact that families go through the process of experiencing grief that may be repeated many times in the lives of the parents of the disabled. While rejecting the term suffering as an aspect of the experience of dealing with the disability of a family member, Renu Singh replaced the term suffering with the notion of a grief cycle, and said: 'I would not call it suffering. What parents experience is a grief cycle. Having a child with disability is like a loss. One may go around the cycle and then come back to it at a later stage'. Singh believes that there are different points in life when the grief cycle starts again because issues keep changing as both the person with disability and parents grow older. There is ample evidence of this throughout the narratives corroborating Naidu's observation that having a special child changes the relationship of the family equations till the family finds their balance again. It does disturb the equilibrium of the family. People perceive that the same social stigma that was attached to disability is now working within the microcosm of the family. Everybody has different reactions to a child who is different. Hence, a new cycle starts every time there is a new stress in the lives of the family or of the person with disability.

Kleinman views this way of suffering as a mode of social experience. The point is not to minimise the seriousness of the problems faced by individual patients, but rather to appreciate the importance that they and their families attribute to the 'interpersonal, relational locus of hardship among the family members. Appreciating the implications eventually requires that we understand suffering as a different way of living illness in the social world' (Kleinman et al. 1995, 1329). Kleinman points out that even within the family, the social experience of suffering is not homogeneous, and it may even be divided.

Similarly, Ghai described parents recounting to her the whole range of emotions they went through before coming to terms with their child's disability. Among the emotions were feelings of powerlessness, helplessness, vulnerability, anger, despair and grief. The experience impacts every aspect of their lives. All of them pass through a series of emotional states before accepting the shock. Very broadly these stages reflect a cycle of initial shock, denial, anger/sadness, adaptation and readaptation. How the sequence of these reactions is coped with depends on the kind of interpretation parents attach to the child's disability. If fate is seen as causing the problem, the chances of parents providing the opportunities for rehabilitation become less. However, if the challenge is accepted, then the endeavour is to put your heart and soul into the child's welfare. For instance, to help new parents deal with the situation, Sanjana's mother talks about how she came to accept the situation herself and 'Now I go about helping and explaining to other parents, building up their confidence to handle the situation'. It is the challenge factor that has spearheaded mothers into setting up facilities for the disabled, not only to help their own children but other children who have similar disabilities, as Poonam Natarajan herself did.

However, a point that was not articulated explicitly and needed more probing was that as the child grows up, the feelings of grief may change to resentment, anger and frustration. These are feelings the parents could not easily articulate: For instance, Chinki's mother (Chinki's mother, interview with the author, Delhi, 2005) said, 'The whole of last week she had an upset stomach because of which one cot got so dirty we had to dismantle and remove it. And yesterday the whole day went in cleaning her clothes'. She spoke in a toned-down manner, 'What to do? I cannot even get angry with her but I got very upset about her condition and had to control my anger. It is not her fault—her condition is such'. Vibha's mother too was not directly able to express her anger towards Vibha, but her body language and voice did give evidence of some level of anger. With some irritation in her voice, she said, 'With such a child our life is over. There is no life for us. I feel strongly that if there is a hostel type place we could send her there'. Naidu gave examples of how in the course of her field experience she had come across parents who referred to their child with disability as a 'headache', or used a term that meant 'waste of food' and denied food to the child with disability.

However, it is also possible that in the case of CP children, since there is a visible physical condition rendering the person incapable of doing any 'productive earning' work, a sense of pity seems to rationalise many of the parents' feelings of anger or frustration about the child's condition. Either way, the parents wish and hope that the child is able to do something to earn a living and be independent; this desire is very strong in all the parents. Initially, all the parents had believed that the condition of their child was not going to be lifelong and all their efforts were directed towards making the child independent and capable of some work or other. Over the years, as the realisation grows about the child's limitations, what parents want more than anything else is that the child should at least be independent enough to take care of his/her routine self-help skills.

An oft-repeated statement of the parents was that initially they did not think that their child's disability was to be a 'lifelong condition', which also emanates from the fact that in normal circumstances it is expected that when children are young they will be cared for by their parents, but when the parents grow old they, in turn, will be cared for by their children. As Dalley put it,

> In the case of the disabled, the caring seems unending and as parents grow older, their caring of the child itself becomes increasingly difficult.... Love, in this context, often becomes fractured, or distorted, by feelings of obligation, burden, and frustration. The prevailing ethos of family-based care suggests that 'normal' tasks are being performed, that roles enacted are straightforward, expected and unproblematic but in reality obligation and willingness are highly relational and context specific. As long as a daughter or son with disability is a child, caring even though arduous falls within the normal parameters. However once the child becomes an adult tensions in the caring relationship may develop: love, obligation, guilt, dislike may all then be intermingled.

In this context, Arun Shourie's book titled *Does He Know a Mother's Heart: How Suffering Refutes Religion* is a moving exploration based on personal experience of the suffering of parents, in particular the mothers of children with disability. Shourie's only child, a son Adit, was born in the US and was diagnosed with CP. After their return to India, Shourie went with Adit to see the well-known philosopher J. Krishnamurti (Krishnaji) at the suggestion of a friend. Initially, he went without his wife. Each time Krishnaji asked that the next time the mother too should come. Finally, all three of them went to see Krishnaji. As the conversation proceeded, Krishnaji talked especially to the mother, probing her feelings with many persistent questions about what she felt about her son. Finally, the mother burst into tears. In Shourie's words:

> Anita, who had not cried even once in the years since Adit's birth, burst into tears. It was as if a missile had pierced a dam. She wept uncontrollably. Krishnaji kept her hand in his, and let her continue crying. 'See' Krishnaji turned to me still holding her hand, 'I told you, you don't know a mother's heart'. (Shourie 2011, 6)

Shourie's critical analysis of religions that begins with his personal experience of watching the sufferings of the family may in part be an expression of his own grief turned into anger at the suffering that God puts children through. It is not easy to accept that suffering; anger and grief are inextricably mixed up. The only difference is that anger is not a socially acceptable emotion for someone who is so totally dependent on others unlike grief, which is regarded as inevitable in the situation that parents are faced with. Grief is then seen as an emotion arising because of the child's as well as the parents' own suffering. Anger must necessarily be turned outward, at God or fate, or the failure of the medical system.

Grieving is a process, and one or both the parents can stop being conscious of it at any point and not proceed to think of it for whatever reason. Further stages of grief may not always be followed in the same order—parents may go back and forth, grieving for their losses while getting on with what needs to be done. Grief is a process that may take a parent's whole life to resolve. Alternatively, it may not even be totally resolved and that is when parents of a child or children with disability live out a life of unresolved grief. Grief may be difficult to acknowledge, but through the narratives and other literature it can be observed that parents of children with disability are *continually* grieving.

A poignant narrative is that of Mohan, where his mother describes the initial reaction to knowing about Mohan's disability. She says

'Then we left our life's boat in God's hands and wherever He wishes to take us with Mohan we are willing to go. So we readied ourselves for the hard work of looking after Mohan'. However, it is important to recognise that the parents' grief is not a sign of failure, inadequacy or self-absorption. Parents, family, friends and therapists and society should expect this grief as inevitable, and it should be recognised and validated. Once the grief is recognised and validated, it becomes a source of growth. After that the parents are able to connect with their personal strengths and limitations, and are able to discover a potential and channelize it in ways that are creative and deeply empathetic.

Anxiety about lifelong dependence on others for persons with disability also takes other forms: The death of a child with disability is an imminent consideration. Even well-meaning people like neighbours and doctors can speak of the death of a person with disability in double-edged ways. Sanjana's neighbour bemoaned the death of her father whose life was valued, and spoke casually about how it should have been Sanjana and not her father who should have died. Another mother of a child with CP referred to the shock of learning that her child was spastic, but being further traumatised by the doctor's remarking that if she were to stop feeding the child, the child would just wither away.

However, another and more common form of the way the imminence of death comes into the lives of the disabled is through the parents' anxiety about their child outliving them—who would then care for the child? In some of the informal conversations with parents of persons with disability, they spoke almost guiltily of their wish that their child should die before them. It is almost as if the parents feel they would be uncaringly 'abandoning' the child, now a young adult, into a cruel and uncaring world if they were to die before the child. At another level, societal pressures of having a child with disability through stigma, social exclusion and non-accessible services underlie the 'burden' of a child with disability that causes great anxiety. In the case of one rural family, the mother described how she had secured her son's future by willing the house and some amount of finances in his name, not in the name of the younger son. The reasoning was that when the younger son's wife comes into the household and realises that the property and money is in his name, she will take care of him and respect him. In addition, he will not be beholden to anyone if the property is in his name.

Another mother from a rural area expressed her anxieties, thus, that her husband often feels that God should relieve Chinki of her suffering soon. The more she grows, the more problems she will have. They are also growing older. Lifting and carrying her is becoming difficult. The other kids are also growing and will have a life of their own. They may move out of this village, go and live in the city and taking Chinki may not be possible.

Even in the case of families belonging to a higher income group, or in a situation where the daughter lives in the US and is supported by the government for services and where her mother has also built up a corpus for her, the anxiety that the mother has for the daughter's future is poignantly articulated in these words: 'I am concerned about her loneliness; she says she will turn loneliness into solitude after I am gone'.

There is another important aspect to lifelong caregiving and burden of anxiety carried by all parents of children with CP, regardless of class. All parents of children with CP, whether they openly express the wish that the child goes before they do or not, invert a strong cultural sentiment of society and of parents whose children, especially sons, die before them. At ritual laments for the dead, in such situations the parents' feelings are articulated with cries such as, 'he was just a child, he had hardly seen the world, he had not even mounted a horse as a groom', and so on; these are sentiments that are shared and the untimely death is bemoaned by all who gather at the funeral. It is, therefore, all the more striking and poignant that in the case of the child with severe disability, the parents want him/her to pass away before them as the situation after them is so uncertain and full of fear of the unknown. The child with disability too shares this fear of the unknown: Among the most poignant words I came across in my interviews are the words of Tejas to his mother: 'Mother you don't die; if you die who will look after me?' Tejas' physical dependence is not the only reason why he wants his mother to be there for him always; she is also his emotional anchor: How can she abandon him to an uncertain world?

How do parents deal with fears for the future in practical terms? Do institutions, society and the state acknowledge these fears and respond to them constructively? From my study, it is clear that while in the urban sector a handful of parents may be able to come together to set up some network for the future caring of their children, this does not seem to be possible for a majority of the parents, especially in the rural and slum areas. In these areas, parents still need to come to terms with the different facets of burden and sense of stigma. For instance, in one slum area there was an old lady who looked after her grandson with the pittance of an old-age pension that she got from the Municipal Councillor's fund. When that money fell short, she used to survive on the charity of some NGOs to give her food. The child's parents had passed away in an accident and she was the only one to look after the child.

For the poor, the battle for everyday survival is compounded by a medical crisis. Alternatively, in case a child requires both special care and some medication to keep the child going, the grief, anxiety and the sense of aloneness, can drive them to despair. It is something I discovered quite accidentally during the course of my fieldwork. I will recount the story as it was told to me by neighbours who had never gotten over the memory of the event that is at the heart of the story:

> There was a family in our neighbourhood that had a child with severe CP. The father worked in a job where he had to spend long hours standing to oversee the work. He used to leave early in the morning and return late in the evening. The mother worked mainly at home since she had two children, and one was a child with disability. However to supplement the income she used to take on some daily wage job. The advantage with the daily wage job was that she did not have to report to duty regularly. With

that money she was able to buy vegetables for that day's meals or milk for the children or purchase the child's medicines since he had severe fits. The father did not get much of an income. Most of it went in paying the rent, and buying rations, and quite a bit went in the transportation to his place of work that was quite far away.

She was a very pleasant person, always had a smile on her face, and managed to bring a smile to others faces. She was very motivated, and mobilised parents to form a parent association for the future welfare of their children with disability. She went from house to house, counselling other mothers especially to come forward and join together. She reasoned that since they are the primary caregivers, they would be best able to decide what kind of future plan should be made for the care of the children.

However, behind her smiling face was a deep sadness. In times of deep depression, she would confide in some of her friends about her troubles. Her husband's job and the stress of looking after the household brought on severe fits, and he would faint at work. This was tough as the employer had started indicating that the family would have to bear the consequences of his losing the job. She had to manage not only the household and the children, but also the husband who was the only regular earning member of the family. The daily looking after of the child with disability was not so much the problem, as was just the daily existence and living.

One day when the father was away, the mother took the extreme step of ending her life. It was a traumatic end, in which even the little child with disability met his end. By the time the neighbours realised that something untoward had happened and contacted the ambulance, and mother and the little child were rushed to hospital, much time was lost. The doctors tried their best to save them. While the mother's condition was critical with not much hope of surviving, the child's condition too seemed to become equally critical. As described by the people around, 'it was as if the child's life was connected to the mother's—just like the umbilical cord is at birth—the cord which gives the baby life seemed to be the cord which also took life away. The child fought valiantly to survive despite his severe disability. But as soon as the mother passed away, life ebbed out of the child within minutes'.

That this account, that I stumbled upon in the course of my fieldwork, should not to be seen in isolation is borne out by a study of disability in Andhra Pradesh. The study reveals that rural families with members who are disabled carry a variety of burdens: social, economic and psychological. There is a pervasive sense of stigma, shame and social isolation. 'Many caregivers spoke of their sense of deep despair and suicide was not infrequently mentioned as a serious option' (Mander 2002, 112). Two case examples show the deep level of despair—one is the case of a mother who had two young children with congenital disabilities. Her husband was an agricultural labourer, the sole family member to bring in money and food. Both parents were desperate and spoke of suicide. Harsh Mander writes that he had rarely met anyone else 'so decisively exiled from hope as that young woman'.

The other is the case of a young mentally challenged woman, who was being cared for by her elderly grandmother. 'The girl's parents had committed suicide as they found the burden of the child with disability too hard to bear amidst their poverty', writes the author. Thereafter, their old mother has fought for many years to keep both bodies alive (Mander 2002, 112).

While it is beginning to be recognised that grief and the 'burden' of care are among the most common problems encountered by parents, Renu Singh states that professionals may not have been able to respond to their feelings: 'We haven't created anything to sustain them', she said. Anxiety about the future of the disabled, which is an enduring aspect of the unarticulated grief of the parents, too is yet to be addressed in a way that could reassure the parents. The continuing grief is also linked to the understanding that the disabled are permanent dependents. While the development of independent living skills is stressed in the West, Singh feels that 'we aren't even working towards it. It will only come about when the movement starts to take it up, when persons with disabilities come together and decide what their future should be rather than us (professionals) trying to decide for them' she says. In a sense, both parents and professionals have tended to regard the disabled as incapable of thinking and acting for themselves—as having no agency. However, as Dalley says, 'Their dependency is not intrinsic to their physical or chronological condition; instead they have been "socially constructed" as dependent because they are arbitrarily ruled out from being party to the bargain or contract which non-dependent individuals are able, or obliged to enter into with society'.

ROLE OF NGOS

Another aspect which emerges from the narratives is that despite the small number of organisations in existence since two and a half decades, the service offered in terms of emotional support are perceived to have been 'tremendous' in the case of those children and parents who could access the organisation. However, over the years it seems that although the number of organisations has grown, the range of services offered has not really diversified. The new organisations coming up still seem to be providing the same basic services—that of early training of the disabled—just as the SSNI and other such organisations had done 20 years ago when they had started the programme. Even organisations such as SSNI, which by now has children in the age group of 20 to 25 years, and can see the changing and growing needs of the children with disability—now young adults—have not, for various reasons, been able to extend the catering of services to this age group.

These organisations have realised the need to change their orientation in terms of the educational and, to an extent, vocational, emotional and social needs of the person with disabilities. Even more so, they have realised the needs of the parents, in order to deal with the requirements of the later stages of the lives of the disabled. Yet there is nothing that they have been able to actually do to serve these needs. This is evident from the oft-repeated refrain of the parents that children with special needs require social interaction and need to be kept occupied.

The parents are caught in a dilemma: They realise that younger children, and children with slightly less severe degrees of disability, can benefit far more from educational and vocational training than they are doing now, as well as the fact that the institutions are constrained by resources and space. Yet the parents also realise, and want organisations also to recognise, that it is beyond the capacities of the parents to be able to organise social and emotional interaction for their children. This is because not only do they lack the resources for organising these sessions, but also because they have run out of the energy that is required to sustain them on an ongoing basis. Their energy is required not only for the physical caring of the child, but also in trying to ensure a secure future for the child once the parents are no more.

Another related aspect is the expectation of support from institutions in dealing with the disabled at different stages of their lives. Since such organisations had come to the aid of so many parents in the initial difficult and troubled years of bringing up a child with disability, therefore, the parents have high expectations from the organisation later on too. In the absence of any other medical or social support structure, the organisation has come to function as a crutch for them. The feeling of betrayal comes across poignantly in the lament of the parents that 'the organisation is not doing much for the children now'.

At this juncture it would be useful to examine, from the viewpoint of the parents, the origins and the entry of the NGOs into the field of disability. About two decades ago, since there was almost nothing being done by the government for the disabled, the parents of children with disability and other concerned citizens in the urban areas found it imperative to take it upon themselves to provide at least some of the necessary services. A few parents and parents' associations have come up since then to cater not only for the early training of children with disability, but also to form a parent support network for the future of their children. Their lobbying for some services which can address the future of the children with disability has resulted in the setting up recently of the National Trust for Persons with CP, mental retardation, autism and multiple handicaps.

One of the services offered by these organisations which has received universal praise is the counselling provided by them. The parents were unanimous about the tremendous help they got from the organisations in the initial years of their coming to terms with their child's disability through counselling sessions, or therapy, through organising *satsangs* or *bhajan* sessions (kinds of religious functions). Such services do cater at one level for the 'felt needs' of the parents; the activities also mark out the capacity for innovativeness on the part of

NGOs, rather than restricting themselves to merely providing services in terms of early training of the child with disability.

COPING WITH DISABILITY

The coping strategies used by the parents to deal with their child's disability vary according to circumstances. In most of the cases, the biggest strength for the parents is each other and then the family support. For instance, in the case of Sundar, the mother was diagnosed with breast cancer, and at the same time, the father's back started paining excruciatingly. Both parents acknowledge that it was the strong family support that helped them to tide over this grim situation.

In the case of Ankur and Samar (Ankur and Samar's mother and grandmother, interview with the author, Delhi, 2005), while coping with disability the parents have financial security since both are working, and are particularly enabled by the fact that the husband has a government job. What helps the mother to go to work is the fact that there is not only a hired caregiver but her mother-in-law is also there to oversee the house and the boys. The mother-in-law in her own way is understanding and supportive. She says,

> We have to support my daughter-in-law also. She did not want to have such difficulties and *dukh* (sorrow). I have never taunted her like typical mothers-in-law saying that it is because of her that the kids are like this. Why should I? Did she ever want to have such children? If we are happy then our next generation will be happy, these kids will be happy. If we fight and cause tension it will have an effect on the kids. The kids understand everything, especially what is being talked negatively about them.

She further tries to cope with the situation through a philosophical understanding and says,

> The future will be shown by 'Him'. What we can do is to feed them and look after them well and lovingly. And we have to do it happily not with despair but as duty. God is helping us; if He wasn't then we could have been in a worse situation. We may have done something in the past for which we owe a debt. For as long as these children are with us we have to

look after them. If someone chastises us then we have to respond to them also. When we take the kids out people look at them and laugh. I give it to them. I say, 'If you can't appreciate them then don't taunt them'. It is with God's help that we have passed so many years of hardship and overcome those hardships. How we have cared for them He is witness to it and no one in society can point fingers at us.

Even in the case of Neerja, she acknowledges that her mother-in-law helped and supported her tremendously. In many of the rural and urban slum areas, support from the extended family appears to be very little. The reasons for people in the slums not having such support could be the lack of physical space to accommodate more relatives in the already cramped space. The reason for not much extended family support is mainly that the other family members also have farm work or related toil to perform, hence they cannot leave those responsibilities. But even in such conditions, grandparents sometimes take the child away to their village; for example, in rural Haryana, Ashok's maternal grandfather took him to his village and looked after him completely without burdening his daughter. She narrates that her father wanted to keep the baby in the village and look after him; he told her that she could have more children, hence, let this one be left with them.

Parental responsibilities are not always shared. Some fathers have helped tremendously throughout the life of the child into adolescence and adulthood, but in some cases, that is not so. For instance, in one case, the father separated from the mother upon the birth of the child with disability (Shankaran). In the case of Amit, the mother said that in the beginning the father helped a lot in looking after him. She described a situation when the two children got a severe attack of measles and there was no hope of their survival. The mother narrates how the doctor had given up on her daughter surviving the attack and the chances of Amit's survival also seemed bleak. The doctor said that if they each drink 5 litres of water that night then there is some chance to save them. Both of the parents left everything, the house was like a hospital with drips and medicines all over. Her husband did not go to work for several days and there was no cooking done, both of them just looked after the kids frantically trying to save them. The two of them immediately got to work, each of them with one kid trying to make them drink 5 litres of water. They had to give it to them with a spoon because they were too ill to sip it. Finally, the night was over, the kids had managed to drink the 5 litres and both the kids survived!

But gradually, the father seems to have got disheartened with Amit's condition and stopped looking after the boy. According to the mother, the father gave up looking after Amit a long time ago, even though he now claims that he cannot do any more for the boy as he himself is getting older.

According to Naidu, field experience as well as research has indicated that in upper middle-class families, mental disability has been found very difficult to accept. This is because there is so much significance attached to 'intellectual' capabilities. Thus, children with motor disability, if they excel academically, are accepted and included into the family relatively more easily than a person with mental disability is. In contrast, in working-class homes, a child with a physical disability is more difficult to manage and is considered a 'burden'. This is because it has been found that children with mental disability are involved a lot in routine domestic chores and help the mother, especially in cleaning the house, washing and collecting firewood. So, by their participation in the labour of the household, they make a tremendous contribution to the domestic economy of the family, whereas children with physical disability are not able to contribute that much in a situation where survival is primary. A child with mental disability can be taken to the field, whereas a child with severe and profound physical disability cannot be carried all that way. As a result, there may be no alternative but to lock up the child with disability at home till the parents come back. Naidu emphatically points out that it is not as if their parents do not love them. They love them very much. Parental love for the child with disability is one thing that has been found across the social classes, Naidu says.

On the issue of whether the child with disability is considered a 'burden', Naidu has found that the child is not referred to as a burden per se but sometimes indirect expressions are used, such as 'He or she is a headache'. In the South, she has come across a particular term which means 'It's a waste feeding him/her' which Naidu feels is one of the most cruel expressions she has heard. There have also been instances when their staff has had to intervene to save the child from dying due to hunger. According to Naidu, the purpose of such an intervention is not a question of passing a moral judgment on the family, because it is a fact that they do not have enough food for the family and one has to understand the situation. But this is also not to say one condones their act, such a situation brings up forcefully the question of survival for everyone in that family.

Parents also seek the support of institutions, but whether the institutions really manage to cater to their demands remains questionable as parents are placed in an unequal relation of power with the institution that provides services to their child. Singh feels that the parents are really not in a position to 'demand' anything from institutions, as they are too vulnerable. Singh cited a parallel instance to highlight the vulnerability of the parents: 'When even we as parents, whose children are not disabled cannot speak our minds out (in making demands) then where is the question of parents with a child with disability demanding anything'. What was being suggested is that the families of the disabled have no bargaining power and are not in a position to make demands from the few institutions that exist.

According to Anita Ghai, coping strategies developed by the family are highly individualised. The strategies depend on the infrastructure the family has. Elaborating the point, Ghai states that any crisis has the potentiality for developing a coping strategy. Thus, there is a requirement for the presence of an existential framework; whenever there is a void of any kind, it also has the potential for growth. 'Whether we grow or not is of course another thing', she points out.

Ghai is convinced that constructions of disability have to change. At the same time, they cannot change unless 'you change and are empowered', that is, having a belief that the disabled can be empowered and, thus, can change. However, for empowerment one would have to create the basic conditions such that empowerment can actually take place. Ghai greatly invests hope in the women's movement and says it is 'feminists who have to create the conditions for empowerment'.

In the context of family strategies used to cope with disability, Poonam Natarajan finds that today parents do not respond in the same way to disability as they did 20 years ago. She attributes this changed scenario to the fact that probably there is more awareness about disability nowadays. The parents probably know that more services are available in terms of choice. She also implies that, therefore, there is less suffering for the parents than before. An aspect to coping that Natarajan has found important is the manner in which the parents themselves handle the child's disability: 'How we as parents respond to the child will influence how others respond to the child', she says. She has however found that it is only over time, and step by step, that parents learn to cope with the situation of their child's disability.

SEARCH FOR A CURE OR MIRACLE

The search for a cure or miracle is the same across the socio-economic classes. The search ranges from babas to medical interventions. As Neerja puts it, 'I had run from every pillar to every post in search of a cure. I was seeking these kinds of places not only for my solace but also for a probable cure'. Arun Shourie along with his mother took Adit to Sai Baba to be blessed. The mothers from the rural areas and slums of Delhi narrated how they would go to the local *dargah* or have *darshan* of a visiting baba (revered person) in the locality. Even medical interventions are seen as miracles and parents who believe in that feel it is a more rational expression, and that they are not getting tied to hocus-pocus. For instance, Sundar's father still believes that there would be some medical progress that would cure his son. Zeba's sisters, living in rural Haryana, were very closely following the details about the latest research which claims that stem-cell therapy can bring a cure for CP. They were hopeful that the success of this therapy would soon enable their sister to avail of it to address her disability.

FAITH AS SUCCOUR

In the absence of institutional support in coping with disability, whether on a daily basis or on a long-term basis, and in the absence of a miracle cure in the attempt to alleviate suffering, recourse to faith has been an important dimension of the lives of the parents. Thus, watching the suffering of the disabled, and the suffering experienced by the parents on their own account, has led most parents to invoke God or the Almighty as an anchor in their lives. It is God who will 'surely find ways' to look after their child with disability once they are gone. The most common form of dealing with suffering is through belief or faith, and is, thus, expressed in spiritual terms.

This leads us to the understanding that although counselling, rationality and active involvement in the cause of the disabled may support the parents, it is the underlying faith in God, and in *seva*, that ultimately helps the family not only during daily coping but also in dealing with the future anxiety for the child. Faith is also important in cases where the disability of the child, per se, is not perceived as the real issue hampering their lives, but rather other factors such as financial or economic problems, or even problems such as a husband's alcoholism.

One reason the family with a severely disabled member who requires lifelong care often turns to faith as a form of succour, is that the state did not seem to exist at all as a support for the disabled. All the narratives reflect this understanding. In almost all the cases, the parents did not seriously or systematically think of the government as an agent or resource that should be involved in the welfare of the disabled. There is general scepticism about the government's role. The common argument is that 'the government does not do enough for the "normal" people, so what is it going to do, or how can it be expected to do anything, for the disabled?'. The only context in which the state or the government appears in the narratives is as an agent of legislative changes; thus, only the parents and organisations which are 'aware' consider that the government can be approached for rendering help, such as reservations, tax concessions or the grant of land for the long-term rehabilitation needs of the disabled. It is this group of parents who have managed to mobilise themselves into a pressure group and demanded services from the government. The possibility that the state should be responsible for the provision of basic medical, rehabilitation and other services for the disabled, including caregiving, did not exist in the perception of most parents of the disabled.

PARENTS WITH MORE THAN ONE CHILD WITH DISABILITY

There were three parents who had two children with CP. In all the three cases, the children were boys and had severe CP. Two of the families belonged to the middle class, while one family belonged to a lower socio-economic level. The profile of the two families belonging to the middle class is as follows: In one case, both the parents were employed, the husband, in fact, had a government job. He had been allotted a government house. The family also had support in the form of a grandmother who oversaw the household while both parents were away at work. They even had a young boy as a caregiver who lived with them and helped to look after the children. The mother was working before marriage and had continued working not only after marriage but even after having two children with severe disability. The mother felt that by her working she was able to supplement the family's income. Apart from that, another major factor for continuing the work was that it gave her time to get out of the situation of being with the children 24 hours a day. She appreciated that respite as healthy because it helped her to avoid depression and also helped in giving quality time to the children. Since she went to work every day, she did not mind not going out over the weekends or socialising, and liked spending it doing housework and being with the children.

In the second family, the mother did not work outside the house. The father had recently set up an electrical goods shop. Although they lived in a joint family, there was not much support for them. They basically had to fend for themselves and look after the children on their own. Since the father did not really have a settled job they were under much financial duress. As a result, the mother had to manage the household within a very tight budget. Although the mother was well educated and was working before her marriage, life had changed for her dramatically after marriage and the birth of the children. Though she felt that she would like to go out to work and supplement the family's income, she feared that if anything untoward happened to the children during her absence, she would be blamed and would never be able to live down the guilt. She had the opportunity to do a course and become a special educator at the organisation where the children went. However, she refused the offer as she did not want to spend all the time just looking after children with disability, at work as well as at home.

The third family was in dire straits as far as finances were concerned. The family of four lived in a cramped physical space of a house which was one long room partitioned by a thin curtain in which the family of four lived. The mother used to run a tailoring shop in the front portion of the room. In between the tailoring, the mother did all the housework as well as looking after both the children who had severe CP. The father was in depression, both because of the condition of the children as well as the fact that he did not have a job. Their financial situation was tough, they just about managed to purchase their rations and pay for the medical expenses of their children, especially the older one who fell ill frequently. The strain on the mother managing all that became too much and she had been on the verge of a breakdown just before the intervention of a local doctor.

In the case of the first two mothers, they openly stated that if they had known that their second child would be disabled, they would have got an abortion done. However, in the third mother's case, she expressed no such feeling except that she had hoped for a normal child. When she discovered that even the second child was disabled, she was very distraught and brought up the issue to the person in charge at the centre, whom she respected a lot. The person in charge told her 'Cry as much as you want today. Look, your younger one is better than your older one, but what if he was worse; would you have thrown him away? Thank God for what you have and live as happily as you can with them'. This gave the mother courage to go on with life.

In the first two cases, both the mothers are well educated and relatively better off financially than the third mother. Yet when it comes to the caring of the children, all three seem to have a unanimous opinion that it is only the family that can take care of such children and no institution would be able to provide the same level of care as the family. In all three cases, if it was not directly stated, it was implied that it is the mother who is the primary caregiver and takes on the burden of care. It is also the mother who is blamed for bearing such children. No matter how much people may say it, in a disguised form it is often implied with that intention. Since the mother is considered responsible, therefore, it is the mother who feels pain and suffering the most.

SINGLE MOTHERS

At the time of the interviews there were six single mothers. Three mothers were widowed (the mothers of Jagan, Jaya and Rekha). Their husbands died of cardiac arrest. One mother was separated and the case for maintenance was still going on (the mother of Shankaran). She belonged to a lower middle-income group. The husband left soon after the child was born as it was known that the child was disabled. Due to the lack of a support structure, the mother was not able to go to work as well as bring up the child. Although she needed her mother's support and her mother did help her, Shankaran's grandmother felt her first priority was looking after the son's family as he was the one financially providing for her.

One mother was divorced (the mother of Guddu). However, since she belonged to the high-income group, she was able to maintain a support structure to help her with the daily looking after of the child, a young adult by now. The presence of the support structure made it possible for her to continue her work and work-related travel.

One mother was not legally divorced, but the couple was living separately (the mother of Surbhi). The reason for the separation was the husband's chronic problem of alcoholism which was having an adverse effect on the family.

In all the cases, the mothers despite their varying income groups and support structures have shown tremendous resilience and strength in looking after their child, now a young adult with disability. They all talk about the difficulty of being a single parent primarily when they have to take decisions on their own. Further, in the cases where the fathers passed away, the mothers have to deal not only with the situation of explaining to the child the loss, but they also have to make up for the absence of a caring parent. In the case of separation and divorce, the bitterness of the situation is often suppressed, and the absence of the father not mentioned.

The role of the institution in providing emotional and psychological support has been tremendous in the case of single mothers. For instance, there is the example of Shankaran's mother who is fighting a case with her husband for maintenance because she is under tremendous financial pressure. She cannot work due to a chronic back condition brought on by the stressful situation. In her case, the organisation has helped by giving her concessions in therapeutic interventions as well as providing pre-vocational training to the child. Apart from that, the mother also does some voluntary work at the organisation for which she gets paid something to manage her daily living.

In the cases of the widowed mothers (of Jaya and Jagan), Jaya's mother, for instance, was a trained senior secondary school teacher before Jaya was born. After Jaya's birth and the discovery that she had CP, the mother stopped working. However, after Jaya joined VS, the mother did the teacher training course and became a special educator at VS. This decision, she feels, helped her significantly in going beyond simply learning how to handle her own daughter. When her husband passed away, it was the organisation that not only provided her financial support, but was also the place which provided interaction with other parents and professionals. Thus, the organisation gave her a social network on which she relied after her husband passed away.

In the case of the other widowed mother (of Jagan), the organisation too has helped her a lot. Since she belonged to the lower-income group, the mother had never expected that the organisation would help her and her son to reach a stage of independence without discrimination. Instead, the organisation gave her the strength and confidence to deal with the child's condition. When her husband passed away, in order to make ends meet, she took up a job as a housemaid. This made it difficult to bring Jagan to VS regularly. Gradually she thought to herself that she would work in the organisation as an ayah and was thereafter employed. This situation relieved her not only in terms of being able to bring Jagan to VS regularly, but it has also given her a sense of security. She also found a community of people with whom she could communicate her problems and a place that helped her find solutions.

In the case of Surbhi's mother, the organisation played a tremendous role in providing psychological support, not just in managing Surbhi but also in coping with the daily stress and ordeal of dealing with her alcoholic and violent husband. The mother says, 'Whatever strength I got to manage the situation is from the help of some of the SSNI staff'.

FATHERS

In many of the cases, the fathers manifest their inability to cope with the situation by either embedding themselves in work outside the house or by going into a depression. For instance, in the cases of both Gudiya and Shyama, the fathers were in a deep depression as a result of not being able to accept the child with disability. In one case, the father had left the family when the child was born and the disability was discovered. In another, the father knew about the child's disability, yet he did not think it important to tell his wife. When she asked him if he knew about the child's condition, he replied that he did, but did not think it important or necessary to share it with her because there would be no point, and being the mother she would only get more anxious and worry about it.

Another mother reports that from the day his father heard about Shakti's condition, he did not recover from the shock. Due to this she had to start looking for a job. On the other hand, in one case the mother reported that when they discovered the child had a disability, she was crying most of the time and feeling helpless about the situation. It was her husband who recovered from the shock earlier. Later, it was he who took the step to go ahead and do the practical things, such as find a school to put him into and start the physiotherapy.

According to Radhika (Radhika, interview with the author, Delhi, 2005), who had worked in an outreach centre, fathers took active interest in their children. She said:

> I've never met a father who would not take an active interest in the development of his child... in terms of exercises or the kind of input that had to be given or finding resources and also managing the household. In fact there was complete restructuring that was taking place compared to other families... fathers were contributing much more to the household... working in the kitchen, cleaning up... I mean completely unimaginable in the Haryana set-up....

For instance, in Chanda's case, the mother narrates that the father is very caring towards the girl. He is always concerned about her well-being and she is uppermost in his list of concerns. He ensures that there is nothing left undone in caring for her. He helps a lot in looking after her. He does not feel ashamed in looking after her. Even if she dirties herself in the middle of the night, it is he who gets up and helps in washing out her soiled clothes and bedclothes. In Vibha's case, ever since the mother started doing tailoring work to supplement the family income, her husband mostly looks after Vibha. He is responsible for activities such as doing the exercises, dropping her and picking her up from the local school or taking her to the doctor.

In many cases, especially in the middle to higher income groups, the fathers play an active role in caregiving. For instance, Neerja talks of the support of her husband who used to oversee all of Guddu's caretaking. This way she could continue working and undertake work-related travel. While most fathers did not talk about being involved in caregiving, one father who has a daughter with a disability observes that despite being conscientious parents, fathers are still not able to come to terms with the situation. He feels that, unlike the mother, the level of daily involvement in the caregiving by fathers is limited; they do not get a cathartic release and so many emotions are just pent up.

THE CHILD AS THE TEACHER AND SUPPORT

Many parents across the different socio-economic groups regard the child with disability as out of the ordinary. For some, the child is acknowledged as a great teacher, even though he/she is still a vulnerable adolescent or young adult, who gives them the strength to go on with patience and fortitude. For instance, Gulbano, who has two sons with CP, says,

> To be very frank my kids are my driving force. My kids have really taught me so many things that I would not have known had I had a normal kid. They have taught me to face life. They have taught me to cope and handle whatever the situation might be.

Neerja puts it in another way:

> You can look at it philosophically. You have to accept life and the fact that you are not the makers of your destiny. And Guddu has done that; he has made all of us much better human beings. God knows whose soul is in him. He is a Rimpoche—he has never cried, he is always smiling and laughing. I don't ever remember I, my husband or my daughter thinking that a tragedy has struck us.

Arun Shourie too expresses a similar sentiment:

> No text or teacher could have taught us that virtue on which Gandhiji placed such significance—*aparigraha*, non-possession—as Adit has. (Shourie 2011, 15)

In some cases, the child with disability is also the emotional support that motivates and gives strength to the parents to continue and not give up. In the case of Surbhi, whose father is an alcoholic and the mother is the one who looks after the children, she says that at moments of extreme tension when the father walks out of the house, it is Surbhi who extends a shoulder for the mother to cry on, consoles her and gives her support to go on and live life. The mother confesses that Surbhi is the emotional anchor in her life, and that makes her go on to face every challenge that comes her way.

NEED FOR A SAVIOUR CHILD

In most of the cases I came across in my research, I found that families had both a normal child and a child with disability. There were three families that had only two children, and both had CP. There were six families that had an only child who had CP. In most of the single-child families, the parents had taken a conscious decision not to have any more children mainly for fear that the second may also be disabled, such as in the case of Jaya, where the disability could have had a genetic reason as the mother had no problems during her pregnancy. Jaya was a full-term baby, and it was a normal delivery and thereafter there were no problems with Jaya such as an illness or a fall that could have led to the development of CP. In the case of Shankaran, the parents were divorced soon after the baby was born. The mother did not remarry; hence, the question of another child did not arise. In the case of Mohan, Naresh, Ravi and Nataraj, the parents consciously did not have another child. In some cases, social and familial pressure did try to force the parents to have another child. In these cases, the hope was that the second child may not be disabled and would help in looking after the child with CP, especially after the demise of the parents. Naresh's mother (Naresh's mother, interview with the author, Delhi, 2005) says that probably if the family had had another child who was 'normal', it would have been nice for Naresh, as the normal child would provide company and would have also helped in other aspects of his development. However, they had no time to think about another one because all the attention was on Naresh. Naresh's mother said, 'No one in the extended family motivated us to have another child, thinking that we should give full attention to this child'.

On the other hand, Mohan's mother narrates that there was a lot of pressure on the parents to have another child. Even so, it was the joint decision of the parents not to have another child because at that time they felt they must serve him only. Many friends and relatives told them to have another child because they believed in the notion of a normal child and they thought it would also help Mohan to interact if there was a normal child around, but the parents were not for it. Today, when they look back they feel their decision was correct. According to the mother, if they did have a normal child their attention would have been divided and they may have even given that child much more attention, better diet, better education, for he would be the one from whom they would have had expectations. The mother philosophically said that it is the expectations from people that make one unhappy. But now 'from him we have no expectation and he is everything for us and we are not dissatisfied with life'.

Ankur and Samar's parents too were pressured by the extended family to have a third child after a gap of some years. Their reasoning was that since there would be such a gap between the second and third child, the latter would not have CP. And it would be this last child who would help look after the two older boys, but the parents were very determined and firm about not taking any more risks and having any more children.

While the above cases deal with the actuality of being pressured to have another child, in Shyama's case no one ever pressured her to have a third child. Nevertheless, she narrated a hopeful dream that she nurtured, of still having a child who is 'normal', and at some level Shyama feels that it will be that child who would perhaps help look after the two children with disability, and that child would also be someone with whom she could just have a normal reciprocal interaction.

SIBLINGS

In the previous section, it can be seen that the notion of having a saviour child in order to look after the child with disability, especially after the parents' demise, was not considered in most cases as an idea by the parents. In cases where there are normal siblings, the expectation from the siblings as care providers of the future after the demise of the parents seemed very bleak. For instance, in Tejas' case the mother says, 'After we die then he can be left in an orphanage. Or maybe these other kids will keep him'. Many of the parents expressed anxiety and doubts about whether the siblings would actually take on the responsibility of the sibling with disability. Many parents were concerned that their other children would go on to lead their own lives, get jobs, shift out of town, get married and have their own families. In Chanda's case, the mother says, 'The other kids are also growing and will have a life of their own. They may move out of this village, go and live in a city and taking Chanda may not be possible'. In Sweety's case, the mother said that it was Sweety who finally decided the bride for the elder brother, as the family believed that then the sister-in-law would respect Sweety and mutually they would have a bond of fondness.

Sanjana's mother too expressed the hope that her other children would take responsibility for looking after Sanjana. She feels that it is ultimately the family which can provide the protection and loving care that is needed by someone who is disabled. In Sundar's case, the parents acknowledged the possibility and the hope that his younger brother, who is very fond of Sundar, would look after him, but they were also worried about how he would manage. Somewhere at the back of their minds they were also anxious about the possibility that the younger brother, or his future family, could become resentful of looking after Sundar. What if Sundar was regarded as a 'burden'? What then would be his fate?

In Shakti's case the mother said,

> Our biggest worry is what will happen after us. I don't know how much I can depend on his younger brother to take care of him after us. He will

also have his own life. Soon after his 12th standard he got a scholarship and went off to the US to study and has been there ever since. They have a good relationship and if Laxman is really very fond of Shakti he may look after him, but I can't say.

Vibha's mother too says,

> Hopefully the other kids will help in looking after her in the future. My son is very caring and says he will not leave her alone even after he gets married. We also have full faith that our son will look after her. The younger daughter will not be able to do so because she will go off to her husband's house and we don't know what kind of in-laws she will have.

In some cases, the siblings did talk of looking after their sibling with disability, but most were non-committal at this stage, perhaps because they were too young, still studying or did not want to address the issue as yet. For instance, in Gudiya's case, the anxiety of the parents is compounded by the fact that the older brother is not particularly fond of the sister, at least in their opinion. (I did not have the opportunity to meet the brother because he was away on official work.) However, the brother contributes financially to the home. An instance of his major financial contribution was at the time of Gudiya's treatment and surgery for a broken jaw. In Surbhi's case, the mother has pinned all her hopes of getting out of this grim situation on the help of her son, who studies and simultaneously works. The 17-year-old son realises the tremendous task he has ahead of him in life; he looks a bit unsure but is also resolved about getting out of the family's desperate situation. He was determined to find a good high-paying job after his studies, so that he could take care of both his mother and sister. He even expressed a desire to find a job outside of the city so that the alcoholic father would not come and trouble them.

However, none of the siblings expressed any shame in having a sibling with disability. For instance, in Sanjana's case, the siblings were very vocal that they were not at all ashamed of having Sanjana as a sister. In fact, they were proud to have such a sister because it made them realise that there were also people like her. Sanjana's presence made them more sensitive to others like her in the course of their school and college days.

Describing the relationship of her two sons, Arun's mother said:

> The younger one wants to be a doctor when he grows up to treat his brother and make him all right. They have a good relationship. They play and fight. My husband is very protective towards Arun and gets angry with me that I don't stop them from fighting but I feel too much interference in their relationship is not good. This kind of playful fighting is like therapy for Arun, at least he tries to move his limbs, tries to say something.

The presence of a sibling in any case may work to create a sense of companionship which may or may not exist with others outside the family because of the restricted social interaction of children with disabilities.

Making Sense of the Narratives II

Living with Disability

STANDING UP TO DISABILITY: MOTHERS AS PIONEERS

Disability professionals and activists have acknowledged that women are good problem-solvers. Once they get over the shock and grief of the terrible odds that their children face, it is they who respond to the challenges they are confronted with. We have seen in the previous chapter that in the 1970s and 1980s, CP was almost a new word and even the medical establishment did not know enough about the condition to tell the parents what they could expect for their children. It was not clear how to facilitate the learning that was similar to what other children were learning. To be trained to be as 'independent' as possible, and work with the bodily condition—unique to each individual—to extract from it through physiotherapy the best in terms of learning skills. None of this was available or considered possible even in the big cities of India. Malini Chib describes her own family's experience first in England when Malini went to a special school, and later when they returned to India. She recounted these experiences as told to her by her mother and from her own memory in these words:

> My mother too developed. She stopped weeping. In the early years my father said she would frequently cry but she became stronger as she saw me improve and be handled so effectively with a new approach. My father then helped to persuade her to become a professional ... a special educationist.

She did well and later became one of the finest special educationists in India. (Chib 2011a, 11)

However, after the return to India the family was faced with a crisis. There were no special schools and there was no inclusive education programme in any of the schools. More importantly Malini faced stigmatisation. Malini writes:

> My distress and the trauma of being with people so completely different affected my mother deeply. She had no one to talk to about her grief and became quite distraught ... she became introspective and started questioning what was happening to other children with multiple disabilities.
>
> It was then that the idea of starting up a model of a school based on what she experienced in England dawned on her ... The whole family reacted in a very positive manner and came forward to support the initiative. (Chib, 2011, 17–18)

It is amply evident from the narratives, as well as the field experience of professionals, that there was a complete absence of state support and programmes for the disabled. This was the context for organisations and institutions to come up in the late 1970s and early 1980s. What is striking is that in India many of the organisations for persons with disability, especially in the case of disabilities requiring lifelong care such as CP, autism and mental retardation, have been pioneered by mothers themselves. It is their struggle and resources in terms of initiative, financial support (which came from their savings) and social support for the cause which often began at the level of the family and close friends that gradually took the organisation forward and expanded its own vision. The mothers progressed beyond merely helping their own child to spearheading the larger cause of disability rights. It is mothers who have held up a mirror to the state and forced it to confront its own limitations. Examples of such pioneering mothers are Mithu Alur, founder of ADAPT,[1] Mumbai (formerly the Spastics Society of India), Poonam Natarajan, founder of VS, Chennai, Merry Barua, founder, Action for Autism, New Delhi, Shanti Auluck, founder,

---

[1] http://www.adaptssi.org/history3.html

Muskaan, New Delhi, Shyama Chona founder of Tamana and Ranjana Pandey, founder of Jan Madhyam, New Delhi, among others across the cities of India.

A brief survey of some of these institutions, tracing their histories and their experiences will give us an idea of what these pioneering women have achieved by way of drawing attention to the needs of children excluded from the schooling system in the 1970s and 1980s. Their work continues to be relevant even today, despite the fact that inclusive education has now become something of a slogan.

Able Disabled All People Together (ADAPT)

Mumbai

ADAPT (formerly the Spastics Society of India) was founded by Dr Mithu Alur in 1972. It was the first special school in India for children with CP. At a time when little was known about the developmental implications of CP, Dr Alur set up the first model to offer treatment and education under one roof in Mumbai. The society grew rapidly and the need for teachers and therapists became urgent. Programmes for professional training and capacity-building began, with an emphasis placed on selecting at least half the candidates for training from areas outside the city of Mumbai. The foresight paid off in ADAPT's increased reach. Within a decade, service centres based on the first ADAPT model were established in Kolkata and New Delhi. The society set up branches in Bangalore and Chennai, both of which are independent today.

After providing special services for more than a quarter century, ADAPT embraced a new paradigm. It began an evolutionary shift from special schools to inclusive education.[2]

The Spastics Society, Delhi, was a direct outcome of the work of the Mumbai efforts made by Mithu Alur. Realising that there was an

---

[2] http://www.adaptssi.org/history3.html

extreme shortage of services for children with neuromuscular disorders like CP, a few young women in New Delhi came together in 1978 to form a small special school. Since people with CP were called 'spastics', they called the organisation SSNI.

In 1980, the school (*called CSE—Centre for Special Education*) could cater to only a limited number of children. As awareness grew and the word spread around about the establishment of SSNI, the number of families coming to the institution increased. Parents became tired of the waiting list and the desperation increased. The demand was for more people to help to provide for more services. In response, the SSNI set up a home management programme to help parents, families and other caregivers to look after the needs of people with disability.

In 1981, the SSNI acknowledged that it was not doing enough as its facilities were confined to the urban child in Delhi. The need in the rural areas was also great, and the resources in terms of professionals, space and finances were meagre. The SSNI decided to link up with the primary health centre of the All India Institute of Medical Sciences (AIIMS) in Ballabhgarh, Haryana, and started the rural wing of SSNI. Here they worked not just with CP, but across disabilities—which led to the entire organisation eventually making this shift. It was the first community-based rehabilitation programme in the northern region of India.

Carrying forward the work of the SSNI, an outstation programme was started to try to provide services for families in the northern states who would not otherwise be able to access specialised services. Subsequently, in 1984, the realisation that there were not enough people with skills to work in the field prompted them to start the School of Rehabilitation Sciences where they train special educators and therapists to work in the field of disability. The courses leading to a postgraduate diploma are now recognised by the Rehabilitation Council of India and in 2002–2003 received affiliation to the University of Delhi.

By 1985, the young adolescents of CSE who were no longer able to avail themselves of the services of the special school run by the SSNI were firm in their thinking that they would not sit at home after finishing school. Nevertheless, there was still nothing else available in the society. They demanded opportunities for training and education, leading to the Vishwakarma Adult Training Programme to equip adults with disability. This organisation enabled young adolescents to find the right employment opportunities and also cope with other changing needs they had.

A decade later, many people at the Centre who had been in the special school in some capacity or other began to argue that growing up in a secluded environment did not equip them to face life in a larger society. So, the Centre realised that it had to make its services more relevant and inclusive. Other dimensions were, therefore, added to the work such as integration of children and young adults into schools, colleges, vocational training institutes and open self-employment opportunities.

The organisation also began advocating policy changes. In 1994–1995, the organisation which had always believed in creating awareness and was trying to change legislation and policies played a major role in coordinating with hundreds of NGOs and lobbying with the government to enact the Persons with Disability Act. The group was instrumental in including people with disability in the Census 2001.

The work of the organisation became more outward focused by the mid-1990s: empowerment, inclusion, sustainability, rights and disability as development issues were issues that were new and challenging, and the incorporation of these new themes led to a process of transformation. The first strategy plan, 'Promoting Access' (2000–2005), was based on this new understanding. While trying to avoid the use of the word 'spastic' in its work, the organisation realised the need to move away from being a special school. Worldwide, the movement in the disability field was veering towards inclusion as a strategy. After a lot of introspection, AADI, as it is now called, was formally registered in 2002. The word is from Sanskrit, meaning 'The Beginning'. They see the beginnings of a new direction for themselves. The acronym 'AADI'—Action for Ability Development and Inclusion—not only reflects their new approach to work but also their fresh endeavours that have grown on the foundations of their past, gaining strength and sustenance from their traditions and values. The logo of the dancing individual, symbolising joy and independence, has not changed.

The vision of AADI is of a world in which people with disability are an integral part of society, participating in the community and living life to the fullest, with equitable access to opportunities and services. Their focus is to facilitate enabling environments in the best interest of the child and the adult, thus, ensuring equitable, accessible, quality assured services using a life span approach.

AADI is informed and guided by the needs of people with disability who the institution believes are further marginalised by poverty and gender inequalities. Through its work the organisation hopes to facilitate, nurture and support opportunities for leadership and greater involvement of people with disability in decision-making regarding their own lives and the processes within their community. It also hopes to develop systems and processes to ensure that there is no exclusion, exploitation or stigmatisation of the persons with disability at the levels of policy and its implementation within their community (AADI).

Action for Autism

Autism figured nowhere in the country's discourse on disability when the former journalist Merry Barua gave birth to her autistic son, Neeraj, in 1981. Her journey has been marked by sheer maternal conviction—she expanded the bandwidth of normalcy to engage positively with her child. According to her the early years were tough. Institute after institute failed to understand little Neeraj's situation. Merry moved to the US when Neeraj was 11, convinced he was not getting the support he required.

A course for parents of autistic kids helped her see the communication disorder in a new light. She worked with Neeraj at home for a year, helping him develop a sense of the real world. His violent behaviour abated and the progress led her to share her work with thousands of similarly affected parents. Barua then turned an educator-activist. She wrote extensively in newspapers and started a journal called *Autism News*. In 1994, she started Action for Autism to raise awareness about the condition, setting up Open Door, a school where she taught her son and one more child. She also launched support groups for parents across various cities. Her mantra was simple: train parents to take care of their child.

In the 15 years since she institutionalised her efforts, her organisation has now expanded into the National Centre for Autism and has become a nodal agency for the disorder. It brings together parents, professionals and trainers, while its website maps everything from legal updates to new books on the subject and information on local support groups. 'I set out to create a model that could be replicated. Today, there are at least 50 schools for the autistic in India', she says. Barua's next step is to explore employment avenues and integrate autistic children into mainstream education. A simultaneous project for her is to work towards a teacher-training model that will help teachers understand diversity.

Finally, the real challenge is: what happens to these children once they are adults and their parents are no more? 'There's not a single home for the autistic. I plan to start a residence that'll serve as a model', she says.

Barua's untiring work forced a policy change in 2006, when autism was included in the Disability Act. Her demystifying of the condition has encouraged several schools specifically for autistic children to be set up. In addition, her reaching out to parents has made her an effective support system (*Times of India* 2010). Merry is also trying to create respite services and open a larger institute that can offer temporary residences for outstation parents.

Muskaan

According to Dr Shanti Auluck, Muskaan was started by a group of parents and professionals back in 1982. This group came together over their common concern about the absence of educational and training facilities for children and adults with intellectual disability in India along with proper guidance to their parents. Since then Muskaan has grown into the largest parents' association in this field in northern India. Parents of intellectually disabled children are encouraged to become members of the Parents' Association so that a strong advocacy group is created to represent the interests of intellectually challenged people in various government and non-government forums.

The guiding philosophy is capacity building rather than charity and welfare; Muskaan endeavours to provide the highest possible quality of life to persons with intellectual disability. It works towards empowering the parents through emotional support, counselling, sharing of information and knowledge. Muskaan enables the parents to understand the development and other psychological needs of their child which is essential to facilitate the optimal development of their children. Muskaan believes creating public awareness is important in order to secure a rightful place for the mentally challenged in the society of which they are an intrinsic part.

Vidya Sagar (VS)

When Ishwar Natarajan was born, little did his parents know how dramatically he was to change their lives and those of several others as well! Ishwar was a child with disability—he suffered from CP.

For the Natarajans, shock and sorrow soon turned into courage and hope. A small garage on Arcot Street was the site of the Chennai branch of the Spastics Society of India. From the garage that was home to three spastic children (Ishwar and two others) it has grown into an organisation called VS on Ranjit Road in Kotturpuram, and is now home to more than 150 children, with a team of 130 staff members comprising trainers, social workers and special educators, besides volunteers.

Ishu changed my philosophy of life. He helped me find my vocation. Indeed, he gave both Nattu (as Natarajan was known to all) and me the emotional wherewithal and energy to work in this field', says Poonam Natarajan, chairperson, VS. Today, father and son are no more. Natarajan passed away suddenly following a massive heart attack. He was only 47. Ishwar died at the age of 22, in March 2001, from complications arising out of chest congestion. But he did not give up without a fight. 'He battled it out for 18 days at the hospital. He inspires not just me but everybody here', remarks Poonam.

Poonam switched from academics to special education when she realised that her son was spastic. She worked with the Spastics Society of India in Mumbai and Delhi before setting up the Chennai branch in March 1985. However, she had her own goals.

> I knew more than anything else that it was all about getting together a high-quality team comprising therapists, medical and social workers and, of course, parents. Taking care of spastic children is a labour-intensive exercise. My primary objective was to demystify disability and establish an Indian model of service. I made it a point to have a parents' training project to enable parents understand what cerebral palsy is all about.

The past decade has seen several changes in the field of disability. This change, from a medical model of disability to the social model, means adapting to the environment and accepting the person for what he/she is. 'Earlier spastic children were treated as beneficiaries of charity. Today, they acquire knowledge and skills and participate in social functions like ordinary citizens', she stresses.

VS has pursued the social model and the results are there for all to see. Several of the children study in regular neighbourhood schools and come every day to the centre for physiotherapy. In fact, Poonam feels that the education system itself needs to change.

VS has been working with tribal children too, through Teddy Trust, an NGO based in Thirumangalam in Madurai, and the Social Action Movement to try and rework the regular school curriculum before the children join government schools.

Poonam's focus on training parents, as an individual tool in the disability movement, led her team to establish family and community-based rehabilitation models. Under family-based rehabilitation, the centre trains parents from slums, lower-middle class and upper middle-class homes. The Home Management Project helps parents learn skills to manage their children suffering from CP, mental retardation, learning disabilities, developmental delay, physical disability and behavioural or emotional disorders. There is always a waiting list of 1,000 children wanting to enrol under this scheme.

Through the Community-based Rehabilitation Project, VS reaches out to more than 2,000 children with disability in Tamil Nadu. CSE, another VS model, looks after research and development and the day school. Complementing that model is the Adult Programme that takes care of independent living, non-formal education and job training, and the HRD Project that covers teachers and volunteer training. Students from VS have joined mainstream colleges and pursued various degrees. Under the adult programme, the centre has helped a few find jobs. The centre has also formed three cooperatives for the members to make and sell eco-friendly products.

VS has also been addressing the needs of adults with disability, such as advocacy, inclusion and human rights. Poonam is not a person to be bogged down by reverses, although she herself admits that even an issue like fundraising can physically and mentally drain one's energy. But she draws her strength from her children, her students who have done VS proud. Ummul Khair, Rajiv Rajan and Prabhakar, all former students, have found the ambience at the Centre so stimulating that they now work there, pushing for self-advocacy. It is from the examples set by children like these that dreams take wing. These dreams take inspiration from the graphical lettering of the initials 'V' and 'S' in the VS logo, symbolising hope and the joy of living: living like it is heaven on earth (*The Hindu* 2003).

Tamana

Shyama Chona in an interview says, 'My daughter Tamana was born with cerebral palsy. It pushed me to found an organisation in 1984 to fulfil the dreams of children with special needs and those of their parents. Therapy and counselling for children and their families is essential for optimum adult rehabilitation' (*The Hindu* 2010).

Jan Madhyam

The idea of Jan Madhyam was born on the lawns of Jamia Millia Islamia University, New Delhi. The year was 1980. Jolly Rohatgi, artist, and Ranjana Pandey, puppeteer, were collaborating on a multimedia programme for preschoolers. Puppets, games, music, dance and crafts were woven together to fire a child's creative imagination. The theme was 'Learning is Fun'. The variety of tasks and stimuli highlighted each child's needs and capacities, making areas where the child performed well or poorly apparent.

It was but a natural progression to think of applying the same technique to children with special needs. Using media was one way of drawing out children who appeared dull and unresponsive, more—it emerged—because of isolation and poor communication skills, than because of their disability.

It was the first of many programmes developed in response to a felt need. Over the next few years, Jolly and Ranjana, joined by Gayatri, a dancer, developed a series of programmes for children with special needs. On the way, new issues came to the fore—a lack of services, negative attitudes in the community, the limited resources of poor and rural communities and the changing needs of the growing girl child.

Today, nearly three decades later, Jan Madhyam continues to be a pioneer, addressing the needs of disabled and disadvantaged young women in creative and innovative ways. Jan Madhyam reaches out to the disabled, especially girl children from the marginalised sections of society—the most disadvantaged in terms of rights and opportunities. It believes in equal opportunity to all, irrespective of degrees of functionality, efficiency, ability and/or disability. Jan Madhyam's programme focuses on the creation of an inclusive environment that allows the able and the disabled to work and play together. Jan Madhyam strives to bring people with disability into the mainstream, using different forms of media—puppets, games, music, dance, painting and clay work—as effective tools for mental development and building social relationships (Jan Madhyam).

ACCESSING ORGANISATIONS

Organisations working in the field of disability have a very crucial impact on families of the disabled, especially the parents and the person with disability. Across the different socio-economic classes, the bond with the organisation is very intense as it is the first contact point for the parents which gives them a positive approach. It is the first place that makes parents feel welcome and that they are not 'bad' people simply because they have a child with a disability. It gives them a sense of worth and a life to look forward to. The support which is emotional, social and, at times, financial in the initial years bonds them so strongly that when the child grows up and the organisation starts withdrawing its facilities to them, it causes tremendous psychological setbacks to both parents and the person with disability.

The important role that institutions and organisations play in the lives of the family and child with disability is highlighted in the narratives. The organisation is almost a part of the family, providing support, nurturance and guidance at different points in time as the need grows.

For instance, in the case of the brothers Ankur and Samar, both with CP, the mother recalls that the parents got a lot of support from SSNI and said with great thankfulness that all along their journey it was the support of SSNI that has been their guide.

Neerja, who also found immense support in the initial years of looking after Guddu and understanding his condition, says, 'They have a very dedicated staff. It is an all women run organisation with a lot of people who have dedicated their personal lives, pain, challenge, whatever you may call it, for the cause'.

Sundar's parents were grateful to the Spastics Society for being helpful in the initial years; in the course of their parent counselling sessions the parents were told, almost right in the beginning, that they should not think that there would be a miracle and that their child would become 'normal'. This statement made them change their outlook and they stopped looking for a cure. The counselling at SSNI helped them tremendously in understanding Sunder's situation—that it was going to be a lifelong condition and the fact that his strengths and potential needed to be tapped rather than focusing on what he could not do.

In Surbhi's case, the mother is very grateful to SSNI, for the organisation not only helped the mother deal with an alcoholic husband but also helped her son, when one of the teachers gave free tuitions to her son.

Shyama with two sons with CP is extremely grateful and thankful, especially for the emotional support that SSNI gave them. Apart from the crucial emotional support, which she desperately needed, they taught her how to manage Sonu and Dharam. The counselling sessions also really helped Shyama. The essence of what she was told during those sessions was, 'What had to happen has happened and cannot be undone; we must try to handle these children and work on whatever strengths they have'. These are statements which have remained with her and really helped her in coping with the situation to this day.

In the case of Samina, she herself pursued finding new avenues through great determination, hardship and persistence as she talked to the Director of the Spastics Society (Tamil Nadu) at length about wanting to do something and to become someone and be independent. Finally, the director asked the parents to leave Samina for three months in Chennai so that they could train her in independent living skills. Realising that Samina also had the aptitude for academics, they admitted her into the Open School. Not knowing what to say the parents just said, 'She is your child—do as you like but make her someone worthy. We don't have the resources to do that for her'. It is since that day that Samina has been living in the Spastics Society's premises, pursuing her Open School studies, to become a lawyer and fight for the rights of the disabled.

In the case of Jagan, the mother recalls that people around her used to question why she had to look after a child like him. She did not know how to respond to them and used to feel guilty about having such a child. It was only after she came to VS and interacted with the staff and parents that she gained strength and confidence to bear the situation and ignore such comments. Later on, after her husband passed away, she joined VS as an ayah. She says that VS has been a big support to her not only financially but also emotionally. It gives her a sense of security and she has people with whom she can talk and communicate her problems, and solutions are found to help her.

However, what emerges from the narratives is that it is only families in the urban centres who have benefited vastly from the organisations. The narratives from the rural and slum areas do not explicitly acknowledge the role of the organisation. This further emphasises the skewed nature of services available and access to those services.

Parents of children with disabilities have not shown much faith in institutional care centres, when they were questioned about exploring the option of institutionalisation of the person with disability. In most of the narratives, the parents across the different socio-economic classes are not in favour of leaving the children in an institution for life. For instance, in Chanda's case, on getting information of some organisation being present in the neighbourhood, the parents took her there. But they did not leave her there; seeing the set-up and the neglect of the inmates, they felt she would just die. They brought her back home and have never explored any other place thereafter.

Ashok's mother very strongly expressed her opinion, thus, 'No, I don't trust institutions. Since it was my parents who brought me up I trusted them to look after Ashok or else I would not have given him to them. How can a mother part with her child? No organisation can look after a child as the parents can, no matter how bad the condition of the child may be or how bad the situation for the parents may be'. She cites the example of television where it is shown that no one other than the family can look after the child with disability. In particular, she talks of a film in which Ajay Devgan leaves his younger disabled brother in a hostel and how the brother stops eating and drinking because he feels betrayed by his brother. She emphasises that 'Our concern is about the quality of care that will be provided, especially his toilet needs. An outsider will clean him up for 1 or 2 days at the most; no one likes to do such jobs, only parents can bear to do such a job for life. At the institution they may even torture, beat him up or threaten him because it is difficult to look after such children'.

In the case of Vibha, the mother says, 'We have very different opinions/views. I feel that if there is a hostel-type place we could send her there. But her father thinks differently. His understanding is that here we have one child and are having such difficulty looking after her, in a hostel where there would be many more, what kind of care would they be able to provide?'

Apart from the fact that there are no good institutions, parents also do not seem to have articulated to the government a demand for such a place. The privately run institutions are too expensive for most parents to afford, and those who can afford these feel that they can spend that money and provide a care and support structure at home itself. This can be seen especially in the higher income families which can hire people to take care of the child with disability such as Neerja, Mithu Alur and Arun Shourie. On the part of the disability movement as well as the parents, there is no active movement in the direction of setting up such establishments. However, in some cities there are organisations such as the Cheshire Homes and some parents' organisations that have thought of developing homes and independent living arrangements. It is acknowledged that running these organisations without any state support would be difficult to sustain and, hence, there will always be a chance of them closing down.

Another aspect which emerges from the narratives is that despite the small number of organisations in existence 20–25 years ago, the services offered in terms of emotional support are perceived to have been 'tremendous' in the case of those children and parents who could access the organisation. However, over the years, it seems that though the number of organisations has grown, the range of services offered has not really diversified. The new organisations coming up still seem to be providing the same basic services—mostly early training of the disabled—just as the SSNI and other such organisations had done 20 years ago when they had started the programme. Even organisations like SSNI, which by now has children in the age group of 20 to 25 years, and can see the changing and growing needs of the child with disability, grown up to be a young adult, have not, for various reasons, been able to extend the catering of services to this age group of children. Such organisations have realised the need to change their orientation in terms of the educational and, to an extent, vocational, emotional and social needs of the person with disability, and even more so that of the parents, in order to deal with the needs of the later stages of the lives of the disabled. Yet there is nothing that they have been able to actually do to serve these needs. This is evident from the oft-repeated refrain of the parents that children with special needs require social interaction and need to be kept occupied.

For instance, until a few years ago, Sunder was going to SSNI but on realising that there was nothing much Sunder could do in terms of vocational training the school asked the parents to remove Sunder and make place for another child who would benefit more from the vocational training. The parents had no objection from removing Sunder and making place for another more capable child who would benefit from the training, but what they felt upset about, and found difficult to handle, was that there was no longer a routine for Sunder; more than that there was no interaction with the outside world. At least when Sunder used to go to the SSNI he used to be in the company of people and he really enjoyed his schedule. Now that he is not going to SSNI any more, the parents have put him in a nearby crèche where he goes for a few hours; although there is nothing much he learns at the crèche and the children there are much younger, but going there is an outing for him, which he looks forward to.

The parents are caught in a dilemma: they realise that younger children, and children with slightly less severe degrees of disability, will benefit far more from educational and vocational training than their children might, as well as the fact that the institutions are constrained by resources and space. But the parents also realise, and want organisations also to recognise, that it is beyond the their capacity to be able to organise social and emotional interaction for their children. This is because not only do they lack the resources for organising these sessions but also because they have run out of the energy that is required to sustain them on an ongoing basis. Their energy is required not only for the physical caring of the child, but also in trying to ensure a secure future for the child once the parents are no more. Another aspect related to the expectation of support from institutions in dealing with the disabled at different stages of their lives is the fact that since such organisations had come to the aid of so many parents in the initial difficult and troubled years of bringing up a child with disability, the parents have high expectations from the organisation later on too. For instance, Sanjana's mother talks about the need and importance of social interaction as well as routine for such persons. Such an opportunity is provided only by the organisation. She says that they had once followed a routine, which no longer exists, and now have to spend the rest of their lives at home. The parents/family do not have the resources to engage these children meaningfully at home without the assistance of organisations.

In the absence of any other support structure, medical or social, the organisation has come to function as a crutch for them; the feeling of betrayal comes across poignantly in the lament of the parents that the organisation is not helping them anymore. For instance, in the case of Sweety, the mother narrates that now she no longer goes to the SSNI as the authorities said that other more 'able' students should also get an opportunity. This decision has upset Sweety considerably, and she has become a very embittered person ever since she left the Spastics Society. This anger of hers is something that the family is finding very difficult to deal with.

Corroborating the observation from the narratives, Renu Singh considers that the biggest strength for the parents is family support. Parents also seek the support of institutions but whether the institutions really manage to cater to their demands remains questionable as parents are placed in an unequal relation of power with the institution, which provides services to their child. Singh feels that the parents are really not in a position to 'demand' anything from institutions, as they are too vulnerable.

EDUCATION AND VOCATIONAL TRAINING

In most of the narratives that I collected, the child or person with disability was associated with an organisation for both education and vocational training. The association with the organisation may be in various forms and degrees of involvement. Some were associated to it from childhood till the period of adolescence. In such cases, the child may have been enrolled in the home-based programme or came to the early intervention centre.

For instance, most of the persons interviewed in Delhi as well as Chennai were involved right from the home-based and early intervention programmes. There were some cases in which the child came for the centre-based educational programme and attended till the pre-vocational stage. This was the case in many of the families in urban Delhi and Chennai. There were some cases where the child continued right from the early intervention to centre-based programmes, pre-vocational training and even attended the vocational training course.

Some may have been given placements or may have been helped by the organisation to set up their own source of livelihood, such as a small shop or a PCO after the vocational training and are independent earning members. There were more such cases in urban and semi-rural Delhi and Chennai rather than in the urban slum area. In some cases, particularly in Chennai, the students have come to the organisation for special help and have gone on to pursue an academic career such as doing their Master's or MPhil.

In some cases, mainly in Chennai, the child attended the centre-based educational programme for a while and then shifted to a regular school; however, such children may still come to the centre for some special help. Similarly, a person may be attending college too. In most of these cases, the child or person is pursuing education successfully through the open learning system. For instance, Samina completed her education through the open learning system and is now pursuing her education in law. Similarly, Kartik is pursuing an MPhil in English literature by attending regular college.

EXPERIMENTING WITH INCLUSIVE EDUCATION

While inclusive education is considered to be the ideal education system for both the children with and without disability, the concept is very difficult to implement in an education system that is entrapped in rote learning and a marks-oriented system. The idea that every child has his/her pace of learning is a concept that is still far from gaining acceptance amongst general educators, administrators and policy-makers. There is a general scepticism that including 'disabled' children along with the 'normal' children will ever work out. The wide-ranging concern is that the 'disabled' child will 'slow down' the growth of the 'normal' child.

There is evidence of this from Gudiya's narrative. As she reached the schoolgoing age, her parents initially sent her to a government primary school in the neighbourhood by getting her admission through an 'approach' (influence). They had realised by then that Gudiya was 'not like other children', and they feared that she would be 'caught out' sooner in a private nursery school than in a government school. Besides, a government school fees was all that they could afford. They also reasoned that, generally, children are not thrown out from a government school.

However, by the time Gudiya reached class 2 or 3, the teachers realised that the child was having problems in 'coping' because she could not keep pace with the other children academically. Further, the teachers could not manage her in terms of studies as well as in terms of her 'behaviour'. The final decision regarding taking Gudiya out of school arose when there were objections being raised by other parents about Gudiya going to the same school as their 'normal' children. The teachers claimed that they were incapable of handling the ostracising of a child with disability by the community even as it might be argued that such a child has an equal right, as any other child, to an education.

On the other hand, experience has shown that both children, 'normal' and disabled, gain a lot by interacting with each other. The development of social skills and emotional bonding is enhanced as both categories of children learn to be sensitive. There is noticeable improvement in the physical well-being as well, since students are expected to participate in all activities. Even the academic development is enhanced through peer learning.

Apart from the benefits for both children, there is a lot of growth and development of the regular or mainstream teacher. In a project on inclusive education in the urban slum area of Delhi, where over 3,000 children with various disability types and degree of severity were enrolled in the local municipal corporation primary schools, the feedback in terms of regularity of the child's attendance, dropout rate and academic performance indicated that it is a tough job to ensure follow-up of each child but that is only in the beginning. As the system gets adjusted and attuned to a routine and schedule, the external monitoring can be tapered off.

An important fact that emerged from the project was that while the children with disability required a support structure to enable them to attend school, an equally important need for a support structure was felt by the teachers who had never been given any preservice or in-service training to handle such children. Nonetheless, the teachers did report that the workshops the project had conducted with them did help them significantly. They not only understood the child with disability better but also other children. The training seminars also helped them to see things from a new perspective and improve their own teaching methods and strategies. However, there are very few cases that show evidence of such developments primarily because there are very few children who go to an inclusive set-up and even if they do, they do not go for a sustained period of time. Malini Chib is a prime example who talks about the benefits of an inclusive set-up in her book titled *One Little Finger* (Chib 2011, 29ff). Her example and experience indicates that what is of prime importance is the mindset of both the labels 'disabled' and 'normal'. If children are treated as children or persons rather than being categorised according to their abilities, only then can their capabilities be recognised; otherwise, her concern is that they will be easily overlooked.

Further, while there is an attempt to move towards an inclusive education through legislation, the ground reality shows that there is very little being actually done. There is some recognition and some new provisions for learning disability but there is still no discussion on, or strategies of, including the milder types of various disabilities, let alone the severe types. In the case of the severe types of disabilities, the subjects are not even considered by the education system to be either children or persons.

While educationists are still working out ways to include children with disability into the mainstream schools, the situation with vocational training is also not very bright. This is because after vocational training there is often the question of where the person's skills will be used. That is, there are just not enough organisations which give employment to persons with disabilities. Thus, in the job market such persons are left with not many options; this, in turn, is limiting the ideas with regard to the kinds of vocational training that can be given. Hence, there is a cycle—the kinds of jobs available for persons with disabilities decides the kind of training but not all persons with disability can undergo that training because of various limitations. This means they are left out of the vocational training, which further narrows the vocational options.

Thus, rather than their ability helping them to find a vocation, the demand in the job market orients the type of vocational training they have to undergo for which they may or may not have the physical and mental capability. This is not very different from the kind of situation that even the 'normal' person faces in today's economy where the job market decides what course of study to pursue and those who do not feel competent or interested enough in it are left with very few or no options.

LIVING WITH DISABILITY

Whether a child with CP has been able to access the facilities available for improving the physical skills of the child, or acquire formal learning skills in a special school or become a part of an inclusive education programme, or gain specialised skills in some vocational training, the end of adolescence leads to a new situation for a person impacted by CP. In the 'normal' world, this is the stage when a person tries to find a job, earn a living and then go on to becoming an independent person who no longer requires the care of the adults around her/him. It is also the stage when sexuality is acknowledged and marriage is planned as a channel for expressing that sexuality, and also as a means to reproduce the family structure. But what of those persons who are disabled? Do they transit into adulthood in the same way? Is their sexuality acknowledged? From the accounts of young adults with disability and/or their parents, it is clear that this stage precipitates a new situation which does not easily fit into the schemes for the disabled that some disability activists have been able to open up; it is not even a stage that parents have prepared themselves for. In the section given further, I will draw from my ethnography to explore some of the issues that begin to emerge when the disabled 'child' becomes an adult.

'MY HEART IS NOT DISABLED': THE (IM)POSSIBILITY OF MARRIAGE, FAMILY AND A NEW HOUSEHOLD

In two cases, the person with disability expressed a desire to get married. One case is from rural Haryana, in a lower middle-income family. The boy runs a PCO. His great desire to get married is attributed by the mother to the reasoning that 'It is not just for selfish reasons that he wants to get married. It is partly because he sees the pain I am in and wants someone to come and help me. He cries when he sees me in pain and says, mummy you have done so much for me all your life, what is it that I can do for you?' He also feels that in the future his brother may not care for him but at least his own children will look after him.

Explaining his desire to get married, he says, 'I may be physically disabled but my heart is not disabled, I also have feelings and desires'. The search for a partner has reached a heightened state in his everyday living and is causing him much pain and despair. It is bringing up questions of his worthiness as a human being as well as a man. He wants to prove that he is man enough by getting married and that will earn the goodwill of his father who otherwise scoffs at him. The father has taken to taunting him about his desire to get married by asking him who will want to marry someone who cannot look after himself.

We may note that this young man's father was very supportive and helpful in looking after him, going from hospital to hospital in search of medical help, even working all night to save his life on one occasion. Yet today he challenges the son's manhood as he cannot earn a livelihood and yet aspires to marry and find companionship.

Another boy belonging to a well-educated, middle income family displayed similar emotions: he got very upset when relatives came with marriage proposals for his younger brother. After they went away, Shakti came up to his mother and said, 'What, Ma, they didn't even ask me about marriage? They are only concerned about the younger one's marriage?' It was then that the mother realised that he too had desires: as she put it, 'He will also be having those kinds of feelings. I didn't know how to respond immediately since I was a little taken aback by the question. I replied to him, first you finish your degree then I will look for a girl. Now I tell him to find a job first, then only marriage is possible. Even he understands that he has to have a job first'. This brings to the fore the issue of masculinity and sexuality and the way the two are so normalised in society and how they equally affect the person with disability, but remain unacknowledged by that same society.

However, it may be noted that when girls belonging to the same age group with a similar level of disability and income group were questioned about marriage, they vehemently replied that they would have to first find a job and be independent. Only then would they consider marriage, if at all. Such a response could be a reflection of the fact that girls are less able to express their desires. It could also be that being girls and with a disability, the need for making an identity for themselves is very important to break out of the stereotype of being dependents. For instance, Samina elaborated on the reason for choosing the profession of a lawyer not only to fight for the rights of the disabled but also because a lawyer gets paid well and, therefore, she would be able to support her family as well.

Similarly, another young girl wanted to pursue her cinema studies because she loved films and wanted to make both mainstream films and films on disability issues. However, at present, she is involved in a battle to convince the college principal and the head of the department to take the course, since they were refusing to give her admission to the course on the grounds that she is wheelchair-bound and will not be able to carry the camera around on shoots. Also, it was argued that the course requires a lot of travel and time-bound projects, and the authorities doubted whether she would be able to undertake the pressures of such a course.

Both Malini Chib and Tamana Chona have also talked about the need and importance of girls with disabilities making an identity for themselves so that they are not identified as 'dependent disabled girls'. It is important to note that even in these few cases where questions such as marriage and career were being articulated, it is access to resources, social networks and organisational support that helps in achieving some of the goals of the young adults.

The case of one couple was recounted to me in which the man has CP and is wheelchair-bound, while his wife has polio in the lower limbs and walks with the help of crutches. Both are active in the field of disability rights issues. They travel a lot, campaigning and spreading awareness about disability and the rights of people with disability. In their discussion on the issue of their marriage which they arranged on their own, that is, it was not a conventional arranged marriage, both faced opposition from their respective families, first on grounds of their disability and second from the socially pervasive mindset that rejected the idea that two physically disabled people could actually get married. The couple talked of how much effort it took to convince their families to agree to the marriage. They also said that they themselves had to be strong in order to take such a step. Finally, the two families agreed to the marriage. However, the decision was then taken that the mother of the boy would live with them to help run the house and do the general looking after that would be required. When the question was raised that such a resolution reintroduces the mother as a caregiver and that too for two people who are both adults, the response of the couple was 'Don't parents in a "normal" household also stay with the children, especially with the son, and help in the house? So our situation is no different'.

While the previous case is a unique example of people with disability getting married in India, the majority of the people are not so lucky. Marriage and disability together are considered a taboo. Although there are sometimes cases of marriages among those who are visually challenged, most of the marriages involve a wife who is non-disabled even as the man is disabled. This situation is indicative of the norm of the woman being not only the wife but also the caregiver.

In contrast, the possibility of the woman being disabled and the man being non-disabled was remote. Parents, therefore, reconciled themselves to disabled daughters never finding a partner, sometimes directly saying so and at other times more obliquely referring to it. For example, in expressing his anxiety about the future of his daughter, Gudiya's father referred to the possibility of Gudiya's marriage, but only obliquely. He pointed out that they 'do not want to sell their daughter to the highest bidder' suggesting that without a huge dowry Gudiya's marriage was not going to be possible.

An interesting discussion took place about the disabled being entitled to marriage with a group of young boys and girls who said that it was no doubt difficult but not impossible to get married and carry out household responsibilities. Some even reacted by saying, 'What if they were normal and after marriage became disabled—after all anyone can become disabled can't they? They may not have CP but could get paralyzed, their speech or hearing could be affected ... anything is possible'.

The issue of marriage is closely related to the issue of sexuality. That is, there is both a need for sex and the development of a gender identity separate from a disabled identity. As Malini Chib, herself a person with CP and wheelchair-bound, puts it very clearly:

> The word sex and disability don't go together. Can disabled people have sex? *Tauba-tauba*! A topic best not mentioned. Even though I have been brought up in a Westernised, liberated family and social strata—the topic has rarely been brought up with me. Most people think that disabled people are asexual. Generally disabled people are de-sexualised by doctors, caregivers, friends, family, and in many cases, themselves. Even social workers and special educators do not see the importance of the topic being thrashed out in the open. Instead they infantilise the disabled person making that person the eternal child. They stereotype disabled people as someone to be taken care of.
>
> In India, due to the enormity of the barriers surrounding sexual relationships, disabled people often find it easier to deny their desires. This denial of sexual identity implies that looking for a partner or acknowledging sexuality may make disabled women, in particular, susceptible to being branded.

Disabled men are not as discriminated on this front as much. They still manage to get able-bodied partners. Perhaps because for the most part, in a heterosexual relationship, it is the women who act as nurturers or caretakers—glorified mummies! (Chib 2011b)

The previous observation and articulation highlights the issues raised in the next section.

WOMEN AND DISABILITY

An important aspect of the narratives, especially in the case of girls, is related to their sexuality, although it is not explicitly dwelt upon. In Sanjana's case, the girl faced sexual harassment twice over. Both times the family did not really believe Sanjana, or even try to listen to what she was saying. The latent assumption seems to be that being 'disabled' and 'crippled' Sanjana and others like her will not be desirable and, therefore, the subject of abuse, since they cannot be regarded as attractive as other women. This kind of attitude also suggests that people around Sanjana almost consider her to be 'a non-person'; during the interview, the mother expressed surprise about how Sanjana could realise what was a 'wrong touch' when no one had talked to her about such matters.

It is notable that on the one hand, the parents routinely say that 'the child is very sensitive' and is 'just like any other "normal" person in expressing themselves or having feelings', but in matters of sexuality thinking about 'normal' feelings seems to be difficult for the parents. The mother's attitude of surprise that the disabled person knows something about sexuality without being specifically told about it, raises the question that just because a person is disabled it does not mean that the intuitive capacity to learn or understand is lost. This way of reasoning undermines the sensibilities of the person with disability.

The other extreme of anxiety is precisely a fear of this sexuality and its abuse. Naresh's mother said 'Adolescence! It is a difficult time and managing it is also difficult. I am lucky that I have boy and not a girl. With a girl in this situation there would be more problems'.

The anxiety, as in the case of most parents of girls, arises when the girl is nearing maturity. For instance, in the case of Lalitha, one of the anxieties that the mother shared with me during my session with her was that she would soon be getting mature.

Given that adolescence is a difficult time for girls, in general, Lalitha's mother was concerned about how Lalitha would manage this life transition given her disability. For the caregiver of the dependent daughter, the anxiety is on two counts—the girl herself as well as the caregiver. The first is easier to express, the second more difficult because the mother/caregiver's anxiety might be read as a reaction to the increased burden of care girls would need thereafter.

While many mothers try to train their daughters to manage their menstruation, some take the option of hysterectomy as a way to ease the handling of the sexuality of their daughter. They reason that the hysterectomy has the added benefit of reducing their child's vulnerability to sexual harassment/assault even as the overt rationale given was the difficulty of handling the menstrual cycle. For example, Sweety's mother expressed a sigh of relief that the daughter's 'future was now safe' because of the hysterectomy.

This kind of reasoning was cited in the case of forced sterilisation of girls with intellectual disability in an institution in Maharashtra, where the authorities claimed that 'now the girls would be safe'. Ghai has forcefully pointed out that by merely performing the hysterectomy, the notion that the disabled girl is 'safe' is very wrong. This is because a hysterectomy only 'protects' the girl from getting pregnant but not from being sexually abused. Perhaps, in fact, it makes her even more vulnerable because the perpetrators would feel reassured that the assaults would never be found out. In a recent study on disability in the rural areas, the project found that it was the young disabled women who suffered from routine sexual abuse and experienced the highest level of vulnerability (Mander 2002, 112). It is such routine sexual abuse that it has to be taken up as an issue by both the disability movement and women's movement.

In many of the interactions with women professionals and disabled women, one often came across references to the women's movement. Parallels were drawn between the two movements in terms of the issues raised by the respective movements. However, equally, Anita Ghai also expressed a sense of betrayal by the women's movement for not taking up the cause of disability and, in particular, not addressing the issue of women with disability. She believes that 'the women's movement has marginalised disabled women totally'. Ghai asks, 'If the women's movement could take up issues like the Dalit question then why was disability left out? One reason could be that existential concerns have not come through to them such that the women in the movement may have reacted'. But, she counters, 'How could it come at all if the members of a women's group have a meeting on the third floor and there is no lift? Or if the material of communication is for the sighted and with hearing only?' Ghai recognises that the sense of having been betrayed by the women's movement has arisen because there is a belief that the women's movement fights against all kinds of oppression and so it must support the disability movement too.

Elaborating on the theme of women and disability, Ghai argues that the focus has to be on a kind of understanding that even disabled women are under pressure. 'As a disabled woman you are marginalised on several counts—one because you are a woman; two because you are disabled; then there can be three because you are a poor disabled woman; four because you are a poor Dalit disabled woman, etc.' Thus, what emerges is that there are different levels of marginalisation. Finally, when the different levels multiply with each other, the effect is very alarming and cannot be easily ignored, she says.

Ghai argues further that the whole feminist spirit, especially in the initial years was to go in for autonomy and independence for women as one of the goals of the movement. Yet nowhere was there an understanding that the 'Indian cultural scenario of embeddedness, in which we, disabled women, too are embedded in relationships, in families was a very different way to look at questions of autonomy. Embeddedness would mean something completely different for us disabled women', she points out. The women's movement has not thought of what autonomy can mean for someone whose life is virtually at stake without some help or assistance including daily assistance. Ghai asks, 'How is a feminist discourse going to reconcile with this kind of reality?'

Ghai raises another concern about an issue which has received very little scholarly attention but is much portrayed and emphasised, especially in the media—that of beauty and perfection. 'And you are saying this to people who are not perfect in any case—but who also get these messages strongly', that is, that the only desirable women are those with perfect bodies, 'whether it [the message] is meant for them or not', she says. Feminists need to build this also into their understanding of what the media does to disabled women too, apart from other women who would not fit the stereotype of the 'perfect' woman with regard to such qualities as complexion, height, weight etc.

Ghai also expressed concern about the health needs of women with disabilities who were excluded from discussions of health: 'Even in the area of public health no one, not even the feminists, talk of access of medical care for the disabled. Nowadays there is so much happening on the issue of reproductive health but no group talks of the reproductive health problems of disabled women', she says. Although Ghai sees herself as part of the women's movement, she articulates a strong sense of betrayal and a sense of being 'let down' by the women's movement as well.

As an articulate scholar and a feminist disability rights activist, Ghai's perceptions and observations need to be discussed seriously by the women's movement. She speaks for more than herself in giving voice to many young women like Sanjana, Gudiya and others whose own feelings have no outlet as the culture and condition in which they are placed does not provide them space to express their sexuality. Even Soni who has had a fairly liberal atmosphere to grow up in and now lives in the US is hesitant/unable to talk freely about her sexuality. She has circumscribed her feelings by thinking about 'pure love' which is higher than love expressed in sexual terms. Her mother was more practical saying perhaps the daughter did not want to think about love and marriage because they have not been in the realm of the possible for her so she did not want to 'go there', as she put it. There is a certain poignancy to this understanding because the mother is also aware of her own mortality, and she has already told us that she worries about her daughter being lonely after she is gone.

Making Sense of the Narratives III

Invisible Work, Invisible Women—Caring for the Disabled

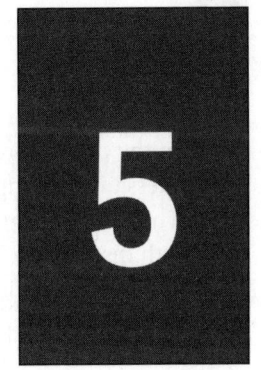

Care is defined with reference to the activities and relations involved in caring for the ill, the disabled, the elderly and the dependent young. It is at one and the same time a form of interpersonal relations and a 'social exigency' or necessary activity in society. Hence, care is particularistic—in the sense that it pertains to intimate human relations and activities—and yet at the same time general—in the sense that it is part of, and integral to, society.

In this chapter an attempt will be made to explore caregiving, specifically the caregiving of the mother of a child with disability extending into adulthood (particularly of those with CP, requiring lifelong caring) in comparison with the caregiving provided by the mother during the course of child rearing, and the professional caregiving provided by nurses. The focus is on the mother of a child with disability through an in-depth analysis of ethnographic material generated in a semi-rural field context and in an urban context already detailed in the chapter on the narratives provided by the families of the disabled. Just as the affective links which form at birth are tied into the mechanical links of servicing and maintenance in the case of healthy children, the same affective links in the case of disabled and chronically dependent family members get tied to lifelong servicing and maintenance functions. In the case of professional care, the function can be limited to just professional 'caring for' without any necessary emotional attachment. This is an important difference that makes the caregiving of the child with disability somewhat unique: The mother of the child with 'normal' abilities provides care to the child for a specified number of years after which the same level of care is no longer required, and the mother can look forward to a time when perhaps the mother's own aging will be supported by the child she is caring for, and the paid caregiving of the nurse is linked to her professional life, the mother of the child who has severe CP is a caregiver for life.

Further, the concept of caregiving is related to an emotional, a physical and a rehabilitative aspects. The disciplines of social work and psychology view caring through a narrow lens emphasising the rehabilitative or emotional aspect. However, if we adopt an interdisciplinary perspective, caregiving is not just confined to 'nursing' or 'looking after', since in chronic lifelong conditions it involves social, economic and emotional aspects all at the same time. With poor institutional facilities and the state's rapid withdrawal from the health and welfare sectors in terms of funding, along with the limitations of the biomedical approach in thinking about disability, caring perforce falls upon the family, and within the family upon women, primarily the mother. For society, the mother of the child with disability is invisible as is her work as a caregiver. Feminists have opened up the field of women's 'invisible' labour, and it is time to do the same with the work of mothers of children with disability, and I shall try to do that on the basis of the narratives that I collected for this study.

THE POLITICS OF SILENCING

In society, caregiving or caring is recognised broadly in two major ways—one is the care at the time of child rearing and the second in old age. Both these types of caring are very different from a non-recognised type of caring—that is for a child with disability.

Most of the recent literature on caregiving indicates that research in the area of caregiving or care work is concentrated in the area of ageing. The focus is on both formal and informal caregivers in the locations of the home, institutions and other alternative facilities for the aged. The research highlights the growing need for formal care in the present scenario where the joint family system is breaking down, kinship ties are weakening and children who are supposedly the carers of aged parents are seeking alternative solutions. Non-institutional care is very dependent on the caregivers within the home, who are primarily women (wife, daughter, daughter-in-law, sister, mother, etc.); even in the formal or semi-formal set-ups (ashrams, etc.), it is women, who are not necessarily professional nurses, who provide the care required by the elderly.

The international trend of an increasingly aged population, especially in developed countries has also led to an increase in research on and development of facilities for the aged; it has also led to an extension in the role definition of the professional nurse as the formal caregiver. Although the nurse as a caregiver is professionally trained, she is also supposed to be caring and gentle, to be like a family member and yet keep her emotions under control unlike women within the family. The underlying philosophy for the nursing profession is to do caring work 'for the love of it', apart from it being a paid job so that it remains a lower paid profession in relation to other types of skilled work. The expansion of nursing as a profession within the expansion of the medical system has led to research in the area of remuneration and benefits for nurses, ways and methods to deal with caregiver stress in nurses and also, its regional and social basis of recruitment, especially in India (*International Labour Review* 2010; Razavi and Staab 2012).

It is not surprising that the research on care or caregiving in the context of the child/person with disability is almost negligible because it is related to the larger political economy and the manner in which disability is perceived as making no contribution to society in economic terms. Thus, while investment in a 'healthy' child is taken care of by society and policies of the country from the time a child is born, the birth of a child with disability is seen as devastation for not just the parents but also for the state, which does not have any supportive policies for such a child or such a family. Scholars have, therefore, argued that 'there is a clear relationship between prevailing social structures, dominant ideology and the way society handles its "deviants"' (Abbot and Sapsford 1987, 7).

Research also indicates that while there is little effort to understand disability as an experience, there is even less research on the needs (social, economic and emotional) of the family of the disabled. Thus, in the context of disability, there are hardly any services provided by the state. There are about 20–30 million persons with disability (2.1 per cent of the population) in India, according to the official statistics, while the figure is considered to be about 50–60 million persons with disability, according to unofficial statistics. This means that the quantum of disability is not confined to the aforementioned figures but that figure multiplied by the number of family members of that person with disability because disability affects not just the person but the entire family.

THE CONTEXTS OF CAREGIVING

Since the fundamental and integral part of looking after anyone, whether he/she is a child, an aged person or a child with disability, is caring, it is important to understand the contexts of caregiving. The organisation of caring in a given society is closely linked to the way in which the society organises different aspects of social relations. According to Gillian Dalley, within the context of the family under normal circumstances, responsibility for fulfilling the caring, nurturing function in relation to the rearing of children and the servicing of adult family members falls upon women (Dalley 1998). Women are also expected in 'extra-normal' circumstances to care for the chronically dependent (the disabled and elderly) persons. As there is relatively little specialised division of labour in traditional societies, caring becomes absorbed into a larger collective if none of the functions is demarcated by a public–private dichotomy.

Dalley further suggests that what has been termed the social construction of dependency is of a different order in such societies as compared to its capitalist construction. In the latter, those who cannot work (for wages) due to physical or mental impairment, or those who have passed beyond the age limit imposed by society on the end of working life, automatically become dependent either on the state or on the family. She also argues that their dependency is not intrinsic to their physical or chronological condition but instead they have been 'socially constructed' as dependent. Hence, systems of support and care may vary according to the degree to which the confinements of the disabled are compounded by the social constraints of marginalisation and stigmatisation, or mitigated by the social supports of integration. In societies which do not have formal segregated care systems, the principal structure of kinship provides the basis for caring. She further states that in situations where society takes on responsibility for providing care, the form of care adopted has tended to be modelled closely on the familial model.

The previous argument probably explains why most national and international research on caregiving is increasingly focused on the aged. The aged are viewed as people who had contributed to the nation's economy and, hence, have a right to state policies to support them in their old age. In contrast, a person with a disability is viewed as a non-contributing entity, in fact, a 'burden' on the state's resources as the person will never contribute economically to society and, hence, hardly deserves any support. The family of such a person is also consigned to the realms of a 'non-entity', almost as a punishment for having produced such a non-productive child. This larger view is internalised by the parents to such an extent that they too have no expectations from the state to provide them any support. In my research I found that when the parents were asked the question, 'What kind of support would you expect from the government to help with the care required for your child?' the answer was preceded by an expression of surprise that parents could even think about such an expectation. Almost inevitably the answer would be 'What can the government do? We are the parents and only we will have to look after them'. But when I persisted, asking, 'Would it not have helped if you had got some help in terms of caretaking support from the government?' The response would be, 'It is our child, and only we will be able to look after him/her properly; no person other than the parent can do the job of looking after children with severe disabilities, because no one will do it with feeling or care!' One mother responded, 'Since looking after "such a person" is considered "*ganda kaam*" (filthy work) by society, parents are the best caregivers'.

Except for very well-off families, paid help for care of the disabled that mothers might be able draw upon is not available. Since hired caregivers are themselves not well off, they accept care work in the households of those who are in the position to contract out all or some of their care work. This is true in the case of families with a child with disability. However, since disability is often associated with stigma while old age is not, professional or formal caregiving for older people is easier to find than help for children with disability requiring intensive care. Trained staff to care for children with special needs are not available in the way such help is beginning to be available to handle care for the elderly. Thus, it is not surprising that it is rarely someone else apart from the mother who looks after the child with disability.

The internalisation of the low value of the work that caregiving for the child with disability actually entails is also compounded by unconscious notions of guilt/karma working itself out which each individual family must bear with fortitude.

CARING AND CAREGIVING

When parents learn that their child has a disability or chronic illness, they begin a journey that is filled with strong emotions, difficult choices, interactions with many professionals and an ongoing need for information and services. The narratives also show that the burden of caring falls on the family, and within the family more specifically on the mother, as stated earlier. This continuous responsibility, in the absence of any formal support networks, has many negative consequences for caregivers, including the suppression of feelings like not wanting to do it 'any more'. For instance, even though Shyama's husband is supportive, he does not actually do the exercises with his two disabled sons because he feels that there 'is no point', as there is no apparent improvement in their condition. While Shyama also has similar feelings, she still goes ahead with the regime reasoning that 'it is our duty to do them'. As a woman and a mother, the option of not doing so does not arise. Similarly, Mohan's mother thought that if she went to work, it would mean that her child with disability would be neglected. She has internalised her commitment to do *seva* to her son to the extent that she says that she is willing to look after '10 such children'. The reality, however, is that in the absence of familial support, Mohan's mother gave up on her dream of becoming a teacher because she felt that her child's needs were more important than her own desire for independence and creativity.

Whenever support from the extended family is available, it has been of tremendous help to the immediate family of the child with disability, especially during difficult times. In Sanjana's case, however, there was no support from either the mother's natal or marital family. Families of interviewees fortunate enough to get ongoing support from AADI highlight the urgent need for outside support services. The model of family support or family-like caring is an aspect of societies and states which have few institutional facilities.

In India, institutional care is almost totally absent; so, when the responsibility for providing care falls on 'society', the form of care adopted is either modelled closely on the family or falls upon individual families directly.

In the absence of support services, the hardship families have to undergo is enormous. They are often not in a position to access outside help due to several reasons. First, they face financial constraints. Second, even though it is specialised work, it is difficult to find persons willing to take on care work, not only because it is underpaid but also because it is considered menial and degrading. Even in families where finances were not a constraint, as in Sunder's case, the service was not reliable and the turnover of helpers very high.

Another interesting observation emerging from the narratives is that despite the small number of organisations for the disabled in existence two to three decades ago, the services offered, especially emotional support, are perceived to have been tremendous by persons with disability and their families who had the opportunity to access them. Even though the number of such organisations has grown over the years, their services have not diversified. The new organisations also continue to provide the same basic services that AADI and other organisations had provided when they started their programmes. Even though these organisations now have disabled adults and acknowledge their changing needs, they have not been able to develop support services to address the educational, vocational, psychological and social needs of this group and their families. This is evident from the refrain of parents that children with special needs require opportunities for social interaction and activities to keep them occupied. The parents are caught in a dilemma: They realise that at some point their wards have to make way for other children with disability to avail themselves of the services of the organisations in a situation of resource constraint, but they also want the organisations to recognise that it is not possible for them to address all the needs of their adult offspring on their own. They are exhausted by the ongoing physical care and apprehensions for the child's future. Since organisations like AADI had played a critical role in supporting them in the initial difficult years of bringing up the child, they are not only dependent on the organisations for concrete medical and social assistance, but they also have high expectations from them. Consequently, there is a sense of betrayal manifested in the lament that 'the organisation is not doing much for the children now'. Indeed, the question is whether institutions can cater for the multiple felt needs of persons with disability and their families. Given the meagre facilities in the disability sector, there is a long way to go as far as meeting all the felt needs of this marginalised group is concerned.

'SOCIAL' SUPPORT

A noticeable feature of the narratives, which comes prominently to the fore, is the role of the extended family in terms of the various kinds of support they provide to the parents of the disabled. In most cases, it is mainly the mother's side that provides the family support in terms of financial, physical and emotional sustenance for the mother and father. It is the mother's 'burden' that draws her natal family to come into the picture in terms of sharing her labour, or trying to give her some physical relief. From the narratives, it is clear that where the extended family support is present it has been of tremendous help to the immediate family of the child with disability in overcoming difficult moments. On the other hand, the lack of family support can have devastating effects as in the case of the mother with an alcoholic husband who had no support from the in-laws, and whose parents could only support her in a limited way due to constraints of resources. In such cases, the mother was very fortunate in finally finding an institution to support her, thus highlighting the importance and role of and need for support services outside the family. The model of family support or family-like caring is an aspect of societies and states which have few institutional facilities.

The discussion on care highlights the fact that in the absence of support services, the hardship the family has to undergo is enormous. It is also evident from the narratives that in most cases the families were not in a position to hire the services of another person to help in looking after the person with disability. For instance, Mohan's mother, in expressing her anxiety about who would look after him after the parents are no more, said that it would be better if they all die together because no one would look after Mohan with the same care and affection as the parents since looking after 'such' persons is considered demeaning. Even in families where they can afford to hire services, as in Sunder's case, the service is not very reliable and the turnover is very high. In any case the inability to hire services is mainly due to lack of finances to buy the requisite services. This brings out the existential fact of the 'burden' on parents in terms of caregiving and raises the issue of poverty, stable and remunerative employment and social support. For instance, in Samina's mother's case, the family needed the finances for just the daily running of the household expenses; the mother *had* to go out to work and she could only do this by locking Samina up for about 6–7 hours every day. This had an adverse effect upon Samina whose legs then started getting locked, neutralising the mother's efforts of exercising Samina's legs before going to work. This 'no choice' situation was followed by the blunt statement of the doctor, 'Do you want your daughter or your job?' An even tougher decision followed for the mother, straddling, on one side, the emotional guilt of being uncaring and on the other, the financial imperatives of the family.

The situation of Shyama who has to look after not one but two children with disability is even more desperate: While both parents are struggling to cope with the physical needs of their children, and require help to look after them, they also have to make ends meet. They have to balance the doubled burden of caregiving with earning a living. Their only support, Shyama's mother, can offer her services only for a limited period because she herself is aged and is in need of support. The limited availability of family support to the primary caregivers is also tilted in the direction of the maternal family. Similarly, in Sanjana's case, it is the maternal grandmother who provided the financial support in the initial years of the mother's widowhood. Even in the case of the financially better off family of Neetu, it was the maternal family, specifically the maternal uncle, who insisted that his sister shifted to Delhi from a small town after the death of the husband so that Neetu could go to a special school. Perhaps the mother's family is involved because they are close to the daughter and understand her difficult situation, but perhaps they are drawn in because of the way the mother gets stigmatised for bearing a child with disability and, therefore, the husband's family simply abandons them to their 'fate'. Again, what is interesting is that it is the mother's mother or mother's sister who gets involved in caregiving. It is women who substitute for each other's labour out of affection and a sense of responsibility. Even in Sanjana's case, it was the maternal grandmother who provided financial support in the initial years after her daughter became a widow.

From working with families with disabled members, Naidu has also found that the mother of a child with disability has stronger alliances with her maternal family. Thus, her mother or sister helps out with the child with disability. In most cases, the husband's family rarely provides any support because they think 'All the problem has come from the mother's side'. Over a period of time, Naidu has found that what happens with all the different programmes of the organisation is that they end up giving a lot of information to the mother. This results in the mother's transformation: For example, she learns to come to the institution by bus, learns to handle people's responses. Through all this learning process her world expands. But one does not find the same thing happening with the fathers. The fathers are busy with their own work. They have their own feelings of anger and grief, which considering the way men are socialised, they often do not find ways to express or to give vent to. Therefore, as the woman is becoming more capable of handling her life, she is really becoming independent: mothers, thus, become leaders in their own right at the 'knowledge' level. Naidu feels that over time both parents need to restructure the way they look at disability, which, given the situation, is very hard.

The narratives also underscore the limited family resources and the non-existence of wider support systems for the care of person with disability. One important issue they highlight is that it is not just medical treatment and physical care that persons with disabilities need, but what is equally imperative is a range of support services to be provided to their families in order to be able to cope. The family burden is not just financial in nature—as shown in the case of Sunder, money was not a constraining factor, and yet reliable help was scarce.

CAREGIVER'S HEALTH

The primary caregiver in most of the families across the socio-economic classes is the mother, especially when the child is young. However, as the child grows up and reaches adolescence and young adulthood, the primary caregivers are still the parents. Consequently, in some families, especially in the middle class and higher income groups, paid caregivers are hired to provide services exclusively for the young adult.

While the higher income families generally have hired or paid services available for other household activities, it is also not difficult for them to get help for their child from a young age. And because of their ability to pay well and look after other needs of the hired carers, they manage to retain them over longer periods of time.

However, in the middle-class families which can afford to hire help do so within severe financial constraints. They generally opt for hiring services when the child grows older and difficulties set in like severe back pain through years of lifting the child. However, in many cases due to their limited ability to look after the needs of the hired carer, they often are left without one, as the carers look for other opportunities and better pay. For instance, in Sunder's case, the father had severe back pain and the mother had to undergo treatment for cancer and this situation forced them to hire help. However, they could get only young boys to help. But there was a high turnover as these boys would soon leave for better opportunities. In the case of Ankur and Samar, the parents got a young boy from the village to help. Although the boy is of great help, he too has aspirations to find a better job in the city, get married and have a family. On the other hand, in the higher income group, the families take care of the hired help as their family members; as Neerja puts it, 'It is a reciprocal relationship, they look after Guddu and I look after their children'.

While the hiring of help by those who can afford it contributes to at least the physical well-being of the parents, for those families who cannot afford it, the burden of caring is a lifelong situation. While many of the parents, especially the mother would not acknowledge that caregiving is a burden, they would like to term it as difficult and a matter acceptance of the situation. When questioned about help from the state, many parents felt caregiving facilities are one area where the intervention of government should be present. As one mother put it, 'The "love for my child" argument is fine for doing everything, but at the end of the day even we are humans and our backs also ache and we will also grow old'.

Rajendra was among the few persons I talked to who recognised the fact that in most of the families, it is the mother who bears the maximum burden of caring for the disabled, whether child or adult. He also recognises the importance of respite from such work for the mother's physical and mental well-being as well as for the family. Thus, the Leonard Cheshire organizations have started Respite Care homes where the families can leave the child or person with disability for a period of time. During that period at the Respite Care, the child or person with disability is well looked after and various interventions are done so that there is no regression in the situation of the person when they go back home.

Thus, a crucial lacuna that comes to light as a consequence of the absence of support services for the physical day-to-day caring of the child is that caretaking and caregiving has taken a tremendous toll on the parents, in both physical and psychological terms. The physical toll can be seen in the form of getting severe backache, which was mentioned explicitly in the case of Sunder's father, as well as Ankur's and Sumit's fathers, a consequence of lifting the child all their life. The responsibility of physically lifting the child begins in infancy and continues through adolescence to the present when the child is a young man or woman—well into the twenties—and the parents have to lift the young adult many times a day. The psychological, as distinct from the physical, toll can be seen in the case of Gudiya's father who cannot walk because of the psychosomatic condition brought on by the anxiety about a daughter's future. It is as if he has taken on Gudiya's physical condition upon himself too, and highlights for us the very real physical stress of parents. Apart from 'routinised' ill health of the parents resulting from looking after the children, in other cases of ill health like the instance of the parent who had cancer, there were no support services outside the family on which the mother could rely throughout the period of her treatment. The NGOs cannot address such problems and at the most, they can provide a sympathetic ear. It is to deal with these kinds of situations, as well as many others, that the state can help as it alone has the resources to initiate a wide network of services to help the individual families which are otherwise trapped in their own individual struggles of trying to cope with their existential realities. For example, Shyama pointed to the need for a subsidy from the state which would enable her to employ domestic help to help look after her two disabled sons; without such a subsidy, she cannot afford to hire any help to provide her with some relief.

Long-term institutional care, especially for a person with severe disability, has not been seriously considered in the Indian context. Consequently, support services provided by institutions simply focus on prevention and early detection of disability and training of professionals. The Western model of the 'modern' institution, which can take over the caring functions performed by the family, has not been considered. However, in the case of Erwadi, Tamil Nadu (2001), the inmates of the Erwadi Dargah were chained to their beds and could not escape the flames that engulfed their thatched huts. Their cries for help were ignored by the asylum owners, mistaking them for the usual outbursts of the mentally ill. The Supreme Court took suo motu cognisance of this horrific incident and called for a nationwide review of treatment facilities for the mentally ill, both in the public and private sectors, and the rural study of 41 villages in Andhra Pradesh highlights the need for institutional support for long-term care, especially of persons with severe disability.

Mander has shown how in rural Andhra Pradesh, the disabled are left without food and care for long periods, as families go out to labour. Erwadi also brings out the indigenous variant of the institutional solution to care, linking it to faith and traditional healing, a system existing outside of the state structure. This leads us to think about locating such issues as the rights of the disabled, care and caregiving in a broader political economy and cultural context. Neither from the narratives of persons with disability and their families nor from the secondary writing on disability in India do we get a picture of either the state or alternative traditional structures providing any feasible, humane and acceptable ways of caregiving.

CAREGIVING—THE PERCEPTION OF PERSONS WITH DISABILITY

While most of the persons with disability recognised the efforts of their parents, particularly acknowledging what their mothers had done, when confronted with the question of whether giving care to a person with disability is difficult or a burden, many did not want to answer because probably it is too close to them and, therefore, uncomfortable, as it makes it obvious that they are not 'able-bodied' and 'independent'. Many felt that caring is something which all parents, especially mothers have to do; hence, it is not something that they did specially for them. While those persons who are articulate were able to respond to the question, those who were not able to express their thought left one to wonder what they were thinking.

Another facet of caregiving was highlighted in a seminar introduction by Komal, who was wheelchair-bound due to a spinal injury after an accident. Komal raised the issue that often persons with disability can also be caregivers, and this is an issue which is not addressed in caregiving discussions. For instance, both her mother and she were injured in the motor accident which rendered them both disabled. However, despite her injury and disability, Komal managed the entire looking after of her mother. While this aspect is important, it may be noted that in Komal's case, she had probably been managing various activities of the household as well as undertaking the caregiving role when she had been a 'fully functioning' person before the accident, and after her accident, she continued it without letting her disability become an impediment. She did recognise that caregiving for a person with disability is difficult, being herself dependent on a hired caregiver but did not term it as a 'burden'. Similarly, after a lifetime of looking after her son Adit, Anita Shourie is now ill herself; nevertheless, she still manages the caregiving and household chores from her bed, remaining a tremendous moral and emotional support for her husband in his writing work apart from mothering her son on an everyday basis and through medical crises whenever they hit the parents from time to time (Shourie 2011, 13).

The gendered nature of caregiving is also implicit in the narratives. Although from the parents' responses it appears that both the mother and father are equally involved; in most cases, the mother is a housewife, or has sacrificed her professional ambition to devote herself full time to caregiving. In other instances, financial considerations compel the mother to engage in both earning a livelihood and looking after her child with disability.

TYPES OF CAREGIVING: NURSES, MOTHERS AND MOTHERS OF THE DISABLED

A professional nurse is trained to provide specialised caregiving, a mother of a normal child provides generalised caregiving, women, in general, also provide generalised caregiving, but the mother of a child with disability is in the unique and tough position of playing the combined role of both mother and nurse. She has to not only provide the generalised caregiving for the child but also do the exercises and other training work important for the child with disability. This work is required on a long-term basis with no perceived stage of life when it will end unlike that for a mother of a 'normal' child, who beyond a certain age does not require the intense kind of caregiving and, in fact, looks forward to a time when the child, in turn, will, or would be expected to, look after the parents. The work is also unlike that of a nurse who has fixed hours of work and can move out of the situation of caregiving and literally 'switch off'. For the mother of a child with disability, it is a lifelong role that she must continue doing day after day without a break, unless, of course, her role is substituted for by someone else—in India, almost always the mother's own mother as I was told.

The long-term care provided by mothers of children with disability was recounted to me by the mothers I spoke to. For example, the mother of an 18-year-old girl with severe spasticity, living in a rural area on the outskirts of Delhi, told me that at the time of her marriage, her mother-in-law was bedridden due to paralysis. The daughters of the family had been already married off and, hence, someone was required to take care of the mother-in-law and the marriage of the eldest son was arranged accordingly. About a year after her marriage, she had her first child, a daughter with severe CP. As described by her, the mother-in-law was totally paralysed and could not do anything for herself. From feeding her to attending to her toilet needs, bathing her, she did everything. And the same things were done with the baby, only more often. All her time was spent in looking after the two (of them) along with all the household work. They used to stay in a house on the first floor. At that time, they had land so they also had buffaloes to look after. She especially mentioned that buffaloes are very difficult to take care of. Her day used to start at 4 AM, sometimes earlier, with caring for the buffaloes, cooking the food for the men to take to the land, attending to the mother-in-law as well as the baby. And the day used to get over when all the household work was finished around 12 at night. In winter times it was even tougher.

UNPAID LABOUR, LOST OPPORTUNITIES, FORGOING EARNINGS

In acknowledging the work of caring provided by the primary caregiver, mostly the mother in a nuclear household, especially in the case of a child with disability, it is important to take note not only of the 'costs' of the unpaid labour but also the lost 'opportunity' and the forgone earnings. Due to severe financial constraints of the family, one of the mothers I interviewed started working as a schoolteacher. Given the time constraints, the mother could not manage to take her daughter for exercises at the hospital. Since the father too went out for work, the mother used to lock her daughter up in the house from 9 to 5 as there was no one else to care for her. This resulted in the child's legs getting locked as mentioned earlier. When she was next taken to the Unani hospital, the doctor sternly admonished the mother to choose between her job and her daughter and do the exercises with her on a regular basis. It was a very tough decision for the mother to take because the financial situation was very bad, the family was in debt and the medicines for the child required money. Finally, the mother quit her job and became a full-time caregiver for the girl till she found a special school for the child a few years later.

One mother described her decision to stay home and look after her child with severe CP as one that left the parents with no options: 'We readied ourselves for the hard work of looking after Mohan'. She 'sacrificed' all of her interests; for instance, she had wanted to be a teacher, but she buried that ambition in order to do what she described as *seva* for her child.

One mother with two children with CP expresses her dilemma and says,

> I am educated and can get a good job but I cannot leave my kids. If I take a decision to leave my kids and take a job to improve the financial situation I have to think what effect it will have on the kids and their wellbeing. Also I don't want to feel guilty that I have left the kids just for getting some money. Making and taking the decision of earning, taking care of my kids, handling my family, is what I find difficult. I know that my handling of them and what I am doing for them is fine, they are getting the best of services. It is a very good organisation. Even if I leave them here at the organisation they are going to be safe here. But if something happens then I don't think my family will easily accept it and will say, 'If you had been there it would not have happened'. They will not think that it is because of the kids that she had to take up a job. So I am scared and worried about that if I take a step ahead and take up a job.

Another mother puts it poignantly: 'By having to look after him full time even I have become disabled because I cannot go out and earn. There is only one person earning and 4–5 people to feed, it is tough'.

Similarly, another mother states that she cannot take up even a part-time job because she has to look after her son, Mohsin, especially since he gets severe fits and sometimes several of them in a day.

This was echoed by many other mothers from low income strata, all of whom stated that they could never go to work because then there would be no one to look after the child with disability. But while in the previous cases, the mothers had to forgo their earnings, in the case of Shyama, who has two children, both with severe CP, there was no choice but to earn a living by running a small tailoring shop in her small one room house. But this also means that Shyama never got to go out as his mother worked from home and also managed her caregiving from there.

There are also situations in the rural and semi-rural areas and urban slums where the trip to the primary health centre for a check-up would cost the family a day's wage and the day they would go to the health centre they would also lose that day's wage. The loss would double if the health centre was far away and had to be reached by public transport, and both the parents were required to go in order to negotiate the bus ride. As one mother from the urban slum narrates, going to the government hospital used to be almost a day-long engagement. The parents would have to go early in the morning, getting both kids ready was quite tough, especially in winter. Then the father would have to take the day off. Also it used to be quite expensive because they would have to hire an auto-rickshaw that used to take ₹150 one-way. This meant, in some cases, that the parents then never took the child to the centre, resulting in neglect of the child in terms of training and other facilities/benefits. This situation is poignant as it highlights the marginalisation of the child with disability and the peculiar responsibility of the parents, particularly the mother, for 'not responding' to the child's need. It also highlights the apathetic nature of services provided and no security for the wages lost in the process. In this context, the proposal of the National Trust Act for helping with caregiving seems ludicrous. Natarajan points out that its schemes are hardly going to work. For instance, the National Trust gives money to train caregivers. But after the training, the parents are supposed to pay about ₹1,000 per month to the caregivers. The pertinent question to be answered is how many can actually afford to give a thousand rupees every month?

The need for organised and institutional support systems to care for those with severe and profound disability is highlighted in the narratives. Though most families have tried not to term caregiving a burden but consider it as a duty, which for various reasons can best be done by the parents and no one else. It is important to recognise that this need for support in caring for the disabled is a need which arises out of the situation, no matter what economic group the family belongs to. The need is obviously greater as one goes down the socioeconomic ladder, but there are instances of even families from higher income groups requiring this support, even if they are privately able to provide for it. For instance, the director of Leonard Cheshire, India, Mr Rajendra, talks of how even families from well-off backgrounds have come to them for support in care of their severely or profoundly disabled family member. Many a times the support sought is a request for leaving the child or person with disability for a while and never returning to take them back. Empathising and understanding the situation of the families due to lack of support structures, particularly in the case of families who are not well-off, Mr Rajendra acknowledges that in such families, caregiving becomes a burden which is compounded by the lack of support systems. He says,

> Caregiving is an added work for 24 hours and we have to accept it. We should accept that it is a reality. And we can't say it's their duty—you know it's a condition where we have to live with it.
>
> We can't do away by saying that caring is bad ... or people who don't want to use the word caring, they don't support care and all that. But I still personally believe, having travelled extensively, having gone to the families, having spoken to people, if you ask the family that's what they say—please provide some kind of support to my child, to my family and that's what they expect, nothing else.
>
> So it is a need unmet for a long period of time. There is still a lot of scope to do some work there. Unfortunately hidden under the carpet and superseded by the rights approach, we should go with the rights' approach, but we should also never neglect this particular need of poor families, especially in developing countries.

While many countries have become signatories to the UNCRPD which is based much more on a rights perspective, according to Mr Rajendra 'in the strive towards a rights perspective, the service aspect for the disabled has taken a back seat, it is almost looked down upon'. In his view, cases where people do require lifelong care for members of the family because of their physical and mental condition, the service aspect is being undermined. Rajendra endorses the fight for rights but he also feels strongly that all sections and categories of the disabled should be taken along in the fight for rights. By not fighting for state-supported provision for care services for such severely and profoundly disabled persons, their right to live and life in real terms is being taken way.

Although most of the narratives indicate that most families are not willing to put their child in an institution, they are also not opposed to the idea if they are assured that good quality care will be provided. The families' hesitation is because of various reasons like guilt for 'abandoning' such a child; God has given them this child and it is their duty to do *service,* so how can they even think of putting him/her in an institution given the dismal condition of most institutions which do take in a child with disability. The need for good and reliable institutional support does seem important to allay fears of what will happen to the child once the parents are no more, regardless of the socio-economic group to which they may belong, but is especially acute for those who cannot make provisions for financial or familial support after they are no more. State intervention in this area is, thus, very important. At the moment, while the state has abdicated its responsibility by not providing services, private organizations which have come up to fill some of the void are ironically facing 'harassment' from the state for providing such services. For instance, in the case of the Cheshire Homes, Mr Rajendra said:

> One of the Cheshire home for example was providing support for mostly spinal injured girls, young adults. They neither have the families' support nor do they have any other centre so they have to live there [i.e. at the home]. They have been living there, they are doing some crafts training and selling those products and earning something and they are continuing with that. The Government of India under the grants scheme was providing grants so far, for the last 10 years they were getting it. Suddenly a new rule has come from this ministry of social justice in the government that says that if they're staying in the same home for a long period of time then such people cannot get support. Our argument is: where do they go now? Where do they go, do we throw them out, do we send them [to their

homes], where do we send them? We can't send them out, the Cheshire Home itself needs support. A small financial support was all that the girls were getting but with that they were able to get about 60% of the cost invested but even that is stopped for the last 2–3 years; now the home is not getting any grant.

What happens to those who don't have families, whose families can't afford or are incapable of caring for them or taking them back? That's a big question now amongst all the caring homes. It's unfortunate. If you look back in the sections of the articles in UNCRPD there is a very clear section on social protection where it is clearly stated that such provisions must be made by the state. Such provisions did exist in India but have now been done away with; this is an irony. On the one side we say we want to follow UNCRPD, and on the other side we take out the provisions. This is most unfortunate.

INVISIBLE LABOUR OF INVISIBLE MOTHERS

Assessing how much unpaid care is provided as well as the time required for care is difficult to measure, both because the work often remains invisible to the women doing it and because it overlaps so much with their other domestic work. Yet while the mothering of a child, caring for the sick and old has been recognised as unpaid labour of women and visibilised by feminist research politically and academically, there has been no such visibilisation of the work of the mother of the child with disability which is laborious, intense and lifelong in its nature unlike that in the case of a normal child or caring for the aged. In the case of a mother caring for a child with disability who requires intensive care, as the child grows up and enters adulthood, the work might actually increase.

To sum up, the mother in the majority of cases is the principal caregiver. Feminists have advocated a change in social attitudes, drawing attention to the need to recognise that caring is not the duty or the prerogative of women alone. An interesting observation on the gendered nature of caring was provided by a father of a young Down's syndrome adult. Presenting the flip side of the father's peripheral role in caring, he felt that through the 'process of daily routine caregiving mothers were able to give vent to their emotional distress and emerged more resilient to crisis situations'. By contrast, fathers, bound by stereotypes of masculinity that excluded them from participating in routine care, ended up suffering from depression because they had no cathartic release for their pent-up emotions in care work.

Unfortunately, as of now it appears that it is only the child with disability who acknowledges the labour and the care of the mother. Tejas' mother sums it up for us:

> Looking after him and doing all the housework is very difficult. For instance because of his weak bodily control, he used to and still soils his clothes a lot (even now) and that takes a lot of time cleaning up, which means not only washing him, his clothes, but also the bedclothes he has soiled. This has to be done immediately because we don't have that many clothes for him or bedclothes, so the clothes have to dry quickly in order to be ready for his next change. Before we did not have a toilet in the house but now since we have a toilet in the house it has become a little easier to manage washing the clothes and one does not have to leave the housework pending for some time and go to the community hand pump to get water for washing.
>
> Yes, in the initial years I used to feel very sad and would just sit down and weep often feeling helpless. And even today after so many years I still feel like that at times. I have other normal children but it is only him for whom I really worry. I look at him and think life would have been so different had he been normal—*lamba, jawan aur sundar (tall, young and handsome)*! In such moments he understands my thoughts. It has been a tough journey looking after him and I will continue to do so till death separates us.
>
> Although he does not speak too often he understands everything, and sometimes if he feels like it, he even speaks. He speaks to me and says, 'Mother, you don't die! If *you* die then who will look after me'.

PART 3

PART 3

State, Society and Disability in India

> The state shall, within the limits of its economic capacity and development, make effective provisions for securing the right to work, to education, and to public assistance in cases of unemployment, old age, sickness, and disablement and in other cases of undeserving want.
>
> (Article 41 of the Indian Constitution)

> Within five decades of the conception and inception of the welfare state in India, its boundaries have got blurred.
>
> —Ali Baquer

The Indian Constitution established that people with disabilities are entitled to the same social, economic and political rights and privileges as other citizens of India in the Fundamental Rights and Directive Principles of State Policy. Article 41 of the Constitution is the only article that explicitly mentions disabled people but it appears under Part IV of the Constitution, that is, under the Directive Principles. Unlike Fundamental Rights, these Principles are not directly enforceable through the law even though they are 'fundamental in the governance of the country' (Article 37), and it is the duty of the state to apply these principles in making laws. Article 41 reads: 'the state shall, within limits of its economic capacity and development, make effective provision for securing the right to work, to education and to public assistance in cases of unemployment, old age, sickness and disablement, and in other cases of undeserved want' (Harriss-White

1999, 148). The mandate of the state under Article 41 envisages a comprehensive social security system, which would enable the lives of disabled people to be fulfilled. However, the Constitution did not make any specific legislative provisions about the rehabilitation and total integration of the disabled in society, and there was no law to protect them from discrimination in their daily lives. Moreover, the mere provision in the form of discretionary office memoranda does not guarantee entitlement. Most of the approaches adopted towards disability until 1947 were based on the concept of charity. During the first three Five-Year Plans (1955–1969), the sole support to disabled people comprised of grants-in-aid to NGOs and the establishment of national training institutes. It was in the first Five-Year Plan that an attempt was made to change the emphasis of programmes for the disabled from charity to rehabilitation. The second plan emphasised education and employment with schemes for scholarships and setting up of special employment exchanges for the disabled. In the third plan, the state encouraged development of facilities for vocational training and expansion of employment opportunities for the disabled, and better coordination between public and private organisations. Up to the close of the fourth plan, most of the programmes were curative or ameliorative in nature. From the fifth plan onwards, emphasis has been on the promotion of preventive and developmental services. The later Five-Year Plans encouraged development of facilities for vocational training and job opportunities. The later plans showed how support for the disabled people declined in real terms as social development priorities, programmes and projects emerged. The main thrust of the welfare programmes for the disabled have focused on prevention of disabilities and development of functional skills. Under the Seventh and Eighth Five-Year Plans prevention was stressed upon. However, the number of persons with disability benefiting from such initiatives remained negligible, seen in the context of their total population.

According to Barbara Harriss-White (1999, 25), plan allocations for the disabled population have been pitifully small in India and have increasingly been subsumed under expenditures devoted to general anti-poverty measures. The disabled have been systematically given the go-by. A significant part of Harriss-White's indictment of the Indian state is that there is little in the way of constitutional provision to safeguard the special rights of the disabled, emanating from their special needs.

Perhaps one reason why there was such a slow recognition of the special needs of the disabled was that there was no enumeration of the disabled since the 1931 census, that is, the newly independent nation did not see the disabled as a category because they had been invisibilised in the census until 1981. Ultimately it was the international developments that drew specific attention to the disabled following the declaration of the year 1981 as the international year of the disabled. Then, in the way the international year of women led to the publishing of the Status of Women report in 1976, which, in turn, triggered off the women's movement of the late 1970s and 1980s and raised a host of questions around gender including women's unpaid labour, the disability question too became more visible. Among the questions that were raised was the poor information available on disability because of the failure to enumerate, or enumerate with some seriousness. Thus, enumeration was the first demand which was believed would lead to recognition by the state and society and that, in turn, would lead to policy formulations and other types of interventions which would facilitate the claiming of rights by the disabled.

In the past couple of decades in most countries of the world, there has been a growing realisation that institutional care for the disabled is not entirely suitable for their individual needs, independence and dignity. The institutional model is, therefore, now being replaced by a relentless advocacy for community care. However, the call for community care is not only based on humanitarian considerations but also on the fact that the Western model of institutional care has been found to be too expensive to run in poorer countries like India. Hence, it was the economic considerations that guided both the emergence and decline of institutional care and provided the rationale now for community care which is being persuasively offered as an alternative to institutional care.

One of the major programmes of community care was launched by the UNDP called the community-based rehabilitation (CBR). Einar Helander, who proposed the concept of the CBR, argues that the CBR calls for flexibility on account of social, economic and cultural situations, the circumstances of the disabled and existing services in individual countries, priorities and policies. CBR is defined as 'a strategy for enhancing the quality of life for the disabled people, by providing more equitable opportunities and by promoting and protecting their human rights' (Baquer 1994, 21). The prerequisites for CBR to become a reality have been described as 'full and coordinated involvement of all levels of society' and 'integration of the interventions of all relevant sectors—education, health, legislative, social and vocational—and aims at full representation and empowerment of disabled people' (Baquer 1994, 21). According to Baquer (1994, 21), such an approach favours reducing the role of statutory services as providers, without going into the causes of their failure. Such a model demands little or no growth in public expenditure on services for the disabled and at the same time uses a language of human dignity, participation, involvement, self-help and family support. This approach promises to shift emphasis from 'everything for a few' to 'something for everyone', in terms of being cost effective and comprehensive in coverage, without demanding further commitment of resources from the government; it also does not provide any clarifications about the nature or quality of care.

The WHO spearheaded the CBR in India and made it a popular idea after its successful foray into primary health care (PHC). CBR is one of the major forms of non-institutional rehabilitation service delivery methods. According to Maya and M. J. Thomas (2001, 44), however, today CBR has moved away from being merely a delivery of service to a method of community development. It aims to promote 'community participation' and ownership in programmes, with the active involvement of the persons with disability and their families in all issues of concern to them instead of them being passive recipients. The CBR programme was primarily meant to be a service vehicle for poorly developed countries, with sparse service delivery systems in most of the regions. Significantly, family members of the disabled themselves generally delivered it through home-based interventions and community volunteers using simplified training packages. The original ideology of the CBR was to provide adequate coverage of rehabilitation services to a population with no services, at an affordable cost, in a participatory model, within the given unique circumstances of culture and tradition. However, according to Thomas (1999, 4), the initial surge of donor funds for CBR initiated a set of projects that could not be replicated due to the indifferent attitudes towards documentation and monitoring. Its impact was limited due to a lack of emphasis on results, replication and cost-efficiency, all factors important for sustainability. Further, according to Thomas (1999, 4), in the case of CBR, sustainability does not seem to be a major issue because donors are usually more concerned with the visibility of starting the project in an underdeveloped country rather than seeing them through. Additionally, South Asian governments do not view disability as a priority. With the growing political confusion in many of these countries, and in the absence of collective bargaining power of the disabled people, it is unlikely that the subject of disability will be accorded priority. Governments are not willing to spend large amounts of money on CBR unless they are convinced about its impact.

Yet there are variations in the kinds of CBR programmes in existence. According to M. J. Thomas (1999, 4), for instance, there are home-based services provided by families for their disabled relatives; self-help projects run by the persons with disability themselves; outreach projects run by a rehabilitation institution; and NGO projects run by paid CBR workers. CBR also functions as an ideology, which promotes inclusion of persons with disability in developmental projects or in institutional programmes located in a village (Thomas 1999, 4).

Given this background and the fact that not much documentation is available regarding persons with disability in terms of the presence of a disability movement, the role of the professionals, parents and the disabled themselves, a critical evaluation of policies and legislation for the persons with disability is yet to be undertaken. Hence, in concluding this chapter, an attempt is being made to understand the disability issue in India through discussions with professionals, the persons with disability and parents who are also professionals. Interviews were conducted with six persons working in or involved with the disability sector: Renu Singh, SSNI, Delhi (professional and director); Javed Abidi, National Centre for Promotion of Employment for Disabled Persons (NCPEDP), Delhi (director and disabled activist); Rama Chari, NCPEDP, Delhi; Anuradha Naidu, Council for Advancement of People's Action and Rural Technology (CAPART), Delhi (professional and head of the Disability Unit); Anita Ghai, Delhi University, Delhi (developmental psychologist and disabled activist; and Poonam Natarajan, VS, Chennai (parent, professional and director).

Some of the themes that emerged from the interviews on a wide range of topics pertaining to disability in India are grouped together under a number of different heads in the following section:

Disability awareness: According to Renu Singh, the awareness about disability is more noticeable nowadays because of the media, although even today the real issue of disability continues to remain within the families which are affected. The awareness is yet to reach the wider community level. In her view, the larger society is not sufficiently sensitised. She regards the PWD Act as having a major role in terms of carrying forward this awareness to the community since there is legislation at least today that will generate its own discussion. And since it is the role of the NGOs to ensure its implementation, there will be an increased awareness as the implementation is carried through.

According to Javed Abidi, there is a very definite trend that can be traced with regard to the increased awareness about disability today. The issue-based coverage around disability was never present earlier. All that existed in the past was that there would be the odd event, which might be reported in the newspapers like some minister inaugurating a school, or a home, for the disabled. This trend continued till 1994. From 1994 onwards, the media was contacted to provide more serious coverage because they were not doing much to focus on the disabled. But sadly, the issue of disability still does not get as much attention as women's issues or the environment, or even AIDS, in Abidi's view. On a scale of 1 to 10, he would rate the coverage of the disability issue at 7.5 but only in the English media. In terms of increasing the general awareness in the community, Anuradha Naidu considers that an important factor is the development of certain activities symbolic in nature, which is unifying for the disabled as well as works to convey a message to the masses. Such an example is provided by occasions like celebrating the World Disability Day or observing the Year of the Disabled and so on.

In contrast to the views cited earlier, and perhaps because Poonam Natarajan was a parent of a child with disability (apart from being a professional in the field), she looked at the question of 'awareness' more in terms of medical awareness. In her view, the doctors today are much more informed about disability than they were two decades ago. Consequently, they have found that the number of referrals has increased dramatically over the last decade.

There is a unanimous feeling amongst the various categories of professionals and disabled activists that India never really had a disability movement per se. But there are others who qualify this viewpoint. According to Rama Chari, NCPEDP, the disability movement has not been totally non-existent. For instance, the persons with blindness were a very strong lobby but only for themselves. The 1990s had seen a cross-disability movement emerging.

Defining her understanding of a movement, Renu Singh, SSNI, argued that a movement should be a 'unified thing' and she strongly believes that a disability movement should be headed by persons with disability. The movement has to start from the grassroots level. It has to start with empowerment of persons with disability. Commenting on how the NGOs can be of assistance to the advancement of the movement, she says that NGOs are not only into 'awareness raising' but primarily into service delivery because one has to look at interventions for the persons with disability, first, and awareness raising follows, thereafter—it is a by-product of the delivery. Ultimately it is when services get opened up that all existing barriers like barriers to services and to information begin to break down. We have to 'open society up', for example, through mainstreaming, for sensitisation to actually begin. In her view, there is also a need to move more towards inclusion and to stop building special schools.

According to Anuradha Naidu, CAPART, a disability movement is a question of whether persons with disability have a say in decisions about themselves or not. Institutions are beginning to see the person with disability as a citizen and are trying to build the required needs and programmes to see how they can adapt keeping in mind this shift of perspective. For instance, the SSNI and VS in Chennai have started the CBR model, and Prajna, an organisation which is seeing the need for persons with disability to be organised, is developing on that theme. In Naidu's view, organisations do have a role in the disability movement and see themselves as allies even though they may not be directly involved in the movement. Naidu believes that one cannot really talk of a disability 'movement' as such because a large number of persons have not left their homes, have not had access to facilities and have not entered into the 'public space'. At most they have come to the institution for some kind of training because their family has brought them to it; this is true especially in the case of the multiple handicap person. Therefore, families and professionals who are like minded have a role to play in the disability movement in her view. For instance, persons with disabilities may not be able to advocate rights for themselves, so how would their issues be raised at all if not by the families and other professionals working with them, she queries.

According to Javed Abidi of the NCPEDP, a disabled activist, there was no disability movement before 1994. There was only the movement of the blind persons among the disabled prior to 1994. He considers 1994 as the origin of the disability movement in the true sense because there is now a cross-disability focus. According to Abidi, a basic criterion of a movement is sustainability. He feels that progress is being made and things are being achieved though the movement is only at a nascent stage.

Regarding the role of the non-persons with disability in the disability movement, everyone is of the view that in every sense it should be the persons with disability who should be in the lead. And it would not qualify as a disability movement if the persons with disability were not leading it. According to Abidi, this is where the philosophy of the Disabled Peoples' International's slogan comes in which says, 'nothing about us, without us', that is, decisions cannot be taken about us (the disabled) without our participation or consideration. However, no movement is complete unless it reaches out to others. So, no disability movement would be complete if it did not have the parents, the professionals and just about anybody else. It cannot be just restricted to the persons with disability: according to Abidi, 'a microscopic view that has been prevalent in India is that it is our little island—consisting of the person with disability, their parents and the professionals. But what about the others such as the architects, doctors, designers, and the media?' he questions. Summing up the nature or character of a disability movement in the true sense of the term, he says, 'the disability movement has to be based on cross-disability, sustainability and have a national character to it'.

According to Anita Ghai, an academic who writes about disability and is a disabled activist, there has not been a sustained disability movement in India. At times, there has been an upsurge of activity and one sees a certain collectivity. But if that is to be compared with other movements, 'the way one defines movements—a people's movement at least', she does not think the disability movement can be classified as such. There are many reasons for this situation. Basically, for the disability issue to come to the fore there is a need for a collectivity to emerge, and to show itself: spaces need to open up for the disabled to be able to use them. And spatially she does not think the disabled have had accessibility. So, in the name of a disability movement if a conference to which only 100–150 people manage to come because they have access to some kind of private transport, whom she would call the elite disabled, or who can travel by air, etc., then this is not enough. So many of the disabled are left out because they do not have the same means of even reaching the conference: how then could such a conference be regarded as part of a movement? Thoughtfully she states, 'I'm not very sure in my mind whether I can say that there is a disability movement today—but what is emerging strongly is a disability consciousness'.

Anita Ghai also dwelt on the formation of the Disability Rights Group (DRG). She said that if one were to sketch the DRG historically, one finds that there are different people in it at different times. While this would lead to a lack of continuity, the turnover can be looked at positively too. But her own experience with the DRG is that it is 'male centric, and person centric and urban based'. Expanding on what could be more justifiably regarded as a movement, Ghai argues it is one where a majority of the disabled can at least find a voice, and be a way of bringing their concerns to the fore. She says, 'however, the utopia that is created is scary (of menu's in five-star hotels in Braille, of lifts into aircraft and so on), and it is that utopia that individually we are fighting for'. In reality, however, we are not fighting—there is no fight really going on. A fight has to be a concerted effort, a continuous effort and for everyone. It has to be such that it gets the bare minimum for everyone.

In terms of the relationship between one set of discriminations and another, those working in the field of disability, or experiencing discrimination stemming from their own disability or of those close to them, often compare the disability movement with the women's movement in terms of conceptualising discrimination and strategies adopted for initiating change in policies. At another level, the expectation that existing movements for change and against inequalities and discrimination would actively incorporate disability into their agendas has been belied. Parents of the disabled or the disabled themselves who have participated in movements can suddenly find themselves, and the issues they seek to highlight, abandoned by the movements they had been part of. According to Poonam Natarajan, politically the issue of the disabled has not been taken up by any other movement. The Left does not think that the disabled can be part of a movement like the women's movement, in her understanding; this was explicitly stated to her by a leading woman activist of an established left party.

A deep sense of betrayal is often experienced and ultimately then it is the disabled and those connected with the disabled, who are left to struggle by themselves.

According to Rama Chari, awareness about the rights of the disabled has been emerging more strongly in the last one decade with the disabled people themselves coming to the forefront and talking about their rights. Earlier the disabled were hardly seen in any forum. Even at the governmental level, there was just the Ministry of Welfare which was giving welfare measures to the disabled people. There were a few special schools set up, and the NGO sector came into operation mainly working within a charity framework doing things like distributing wheelchairs. Some provided special education, or therapy or vocational training. Finally, some disabled people felt that there should be some attempts at working in the area of rights. No matter what their disability is and where they are placed, equality and opportunity is important and has to cut across all boundaries, argues Renu Singh.

Javed Abidi describes the history of how the question of rights of the disabled came up as an issue in India. In 1994, some people in the disability sector were upset with what was going on, or rather not happening and that led to the formation of the DRG. It was the first time that an advocacy group was formed and a cross-disability perspective was taken to demand rights for all categories of the disabled. Thus, began the 'fight and demand for the rights of the disabled'. The DRG did work in a systematic way. Since the DRG was not politically affiliated to any party, the group members met with the ministers of the Congress and the BJP regarding rights and policies for the disabled.

Summing up the movement for rights, Anita Ghai argues that based on her own personal experience, she has picked up the position that the 'personal is political'. She is strongly of the opinion that one should work for that particular cause which is going to benefit the maximum number of people. She feels that clarity of vision is lacking in the disability sector in India. She attributes this to the fact that there is not much understanding of disability as a concept. The demands that are being made are just in terms of 'concessions', even if it they are couched in the terminology of rights.

According to Javed Abidi, India is very much a welfare state since India states it more categorically than the US or the European countries. India has a huge number of welfare schemes. However, what is unfortunate, says Abidi, is that disability does not find a place in that welfare frame. In 1995, the resource allocation for the disabled at the central level was ₹470 million. Presuming that at that time the number of disabled was about 50 million, the stated amount works out to ₹9 per disabled person per annum. Abidi angrily asks: Why is it that the resource allocation for the disabled was so low and yet was never questioned by those working in the disability sector. An argument often given is that India is a poor country, but thankfully it is not an answer that is given now. Abidi's explanation for the poor resource allocation for the disabled was that when a minister goes on tour he announces many packages for the people as a political and vote seeking gimmick. Fed up with this game he began to question the ministers by asking them that if there was money for everyone how come there is none for the disabled. The budget of the welfare wing in the early 1990s was about ₹10,000 million out of which the bulk was distributed between the SC/ST and Minorities and the leftover of ₹470 million was given to the disability sector. Abidi says that the answer to his question about why is there no money for the disabled is 'hidden' in the allotment itself; it is because the others are a vote bank, whereas the disabled are not. Since the disabled have never united and fought this injustice, Abidi argues that there is no point in placing the entire blame on others for the low priority being accorded to the disabled. Arguing with the ministers has had some effect and this year the resource allocation for the disabled is somewhere near about ₹10,000 million.

Poonam Natarajan personally believes that the government wants to talk to those who are involved in the field of disability. According to her, people should be willing to do consultancy for the government because it is these people who are working in the field and getting all that 'rich experience' while the policy-makers are bureaucrats who just sit in their offices. According to her, it is very different working with the government now than it was earlier. Today people's field experience does influence bureaucrats and 'they listen to you', she says. They also genuinely want to know what the field situation is because they realise that they do not know what is happening on the ground. For instance, if you tell them that the wheelchairs do not work, or that what the government is making in a certain factory is not working, they close down the production in that factory and go on to planning to make something better. But this is not to state that governments are 'not dumping everything on the NGOs', which they are.

According to Anita Ghai, 'What people do not realise is that the state in its attempt to promote the NGOs is actually giving up its responsibility'. The issue of rights is emerging but she questions, 'for how many?' Rights are not emerging for everybody. According to Ghai, there is an issue-based mode of fight. First, it was the hunger strike to be counted in the census, then demanding air travel concession or income tax reduction or exemption and so on. She considers this to be a 'concessional' approach and not a question of acknowledging rights. According to Ghai, the welfare agendas are not looked into because they do not serve the purpose of those claiming to fight for the 'rights' of the disabled. On the other hand, there are some of the disabled who are allowing themselves to be co-opted by the government which has consequences for the movement as a whole.

Among the most disappointing areas where the state has failed to make an early intervention to alleviate the condition of the child with disability to improve its health, skills, growth and life chance is evident from the exclusion of the child with disability from the Integrated Child Development Services (ICDS) programme. While there is no explicit clause excluding the disabled, in practice this was so because there was no specific provision to address the special needs of the disabled preschool child (Alur 2003, 13). She sees this as a consequence of a lack in conceptual clarity on the part of the state towards the disabled. She writes:

> In the last fifty [now sixty] years since Indian independence no step has been taken to create a uniform policy for child with disability which indicates the strong absence of a political will to do so. (Alur 2003, 214)

Poonam Natarajan also points out that a close look at the ICDS and the Anganwadi project revealed major lacunae in the programmes: for example, the field-level workers should have been trained in handling all children, including the child with disability, to make the programme a more comprehensive and purposeful venture. But instead the Anganwadi workers refer the child with disability to the PHC and nothing more is done to include the child with disability in the programme. Natarajan and a few others have, therefore, been lobbying with the government on the point that since the Anganwadi worker is meant for all children of a particular locality then why should the child with disability be excluded from her purview (Anganwadi workers are generally women).

Similarly, an evaluation of the workings of the District Primary Education Programme (DPEP) schools by Natarajan's organisation revealed that while the DPEP had a component catering to children with special needs, it was found to be very ineffective. Further, the municipal schools which are supposed to take in children with disabilities, in practice send these children to the hospital and thereafter, the state forgets about the child with disability.

Natarajan also pointed out that among the various education programmes, the 'Sarva Shiksha Abhiyan' has allotted ₹1,200 per annum per child with disability. According to Natarajan, this is enough money for any aid or appliance a child with disability needs but the common complaint one continues to encounter is that there is no money; in most cases the money is not the real problem, the issue is actually planning a cost-effective and purposeful utilisation of funds. Natarajan cited the well-meaning example of the collector of Nilgiris who is regarded as one of the most dynamic collectors in the country. With the money from the National Trust, she is setting up homes for special children from the ages of 6 to 16 years with the intention that this measure will help to provide training to the children and that once the training is over, they will go back to the family. The question Natarajan raises is why have homes for training? History reveals that the emphasis of many people in the disability sector the world over, and in India too, has been to work against setting up residential institutions or homes within which the disabled are confined and training is imparted to them away from their families and society. Further, Natarajan points out that even if the reasoning regarding training the children to be independent adults is accepted, sending the children back to the family later is going to be very difficult; they would have become adolescents by the time they finish their training and social adjustment at a later stage becomes much tougher. Hence, Natarajan feels that with this kind of 'mindless' planning going on, we may come back a full circle and probably to a worse scenario considering the amount of time one would have lost in the process. Although the National Trust Act does fund homes, Natarajan thinks that the collectors are not the ones who should set them up. The parents of the disabled and the disabled themselves should decide upon a measure such as this.

In recent years, the new buzzword both in the state and among international and national NGOs is the need for disability programmes to move to the CBR model. Disability activists and professionals reflect this shift. For example, Renu Singh described the process of how the SSNI shifted from a centre based model to a CBR model. The SSNI had started with only CP children. But in retrospect, today, the organisation has realised that they need to move away from this institution-based model to a community-based model. Unknowingly though in the rural programmes even 20 years back the SSNI was looking at all children with disability within the framework of the community because they realised that they had to work with everybody. They found that they could not restrict their work with just one category of people. What they had not realised was that the same framework could be applied in the urban set-up too. But today in the city they are trying to move towards incorporating the disabled into the community, calling it integrated services. The aim is to work towards 'convergence' with the existing structures instead of building new structures, which are segregated. Therefore, they have plans to tie up with a NGO working in the area of development in an urban slum area. The SSNI proposes that no segregation is required and they will offer technical expertise to the NGO, thereby cutting across all disabilities automatically. According to Singh, it is with this kind of thinking that they have grown in their own perception and find that this approach is more holistic.

The majority of the organisations catering to the persons with disability today are institution based, especially the new institutions that are coming up. But the issue that confronts the disability sector is: How many mainstream schools are actually willing to take the disabled into their programme? According to Singh, even the DPEP, Anganwadi and Balwadi projects are really not opening up to include the child with disability. Singh argues that what needs to be carefully examined is what services the programmes are providing to all children, including the child with disability. If public services do not cater to the disabled then such a situation will inevitably lead to special schools coming up. That will be the only alternative for those disabled who are excluded from the public system. Even mainstream schools, which are opening up a section for the disabled, are building up only in terms of resource centres in which there will be special educators. Further, the inclusion of the disabled is only in certain activities of the school not in all of them. Thus, there is no social inclusion at all and so the talk of inclusion by such schools is a just a myth.

According to Singh, what is needed is a sustained support system for the disabled. For this the NGOs, professionals and the disabled, all will have to collaborate. Instead of giving a one-to-one instruction, the need is to give training to the mainstream teachers. Singh feels that in a country like ours, we need to learn from the West, that is, deconstructing the special schools and services they have created. And one needs to work towards convergence. Reflecting on the ultimate aim of any service, Singh cites the following example: some CP persons who pass out with 90 per cent marks from SSNI call themselves 'special school survivors'. This perception exists even after 25 years of providing special services, regarded as excellent service and considered one of the best offered in the country. Singh says,

> the experience has made us rethink our strategies; ultimately at the heart of all this is the person with disability. If that person after all this input is unable to find a place in society, we need to take another look at our strategies and think about how we work through the community. Especially in a country like ours, where there is shortage of resources, working towards inclusion should begin from day one and bring about a change in the general quality of services by catering to the disabled.

Regarding the need for institutions for the severely disabled, Singh feels that there would always be a category, which would require institutions to take care of them, but they are hoping that schools would start including such cases. Singh argues that if one talks of education for all, 'Sarva Shiksha Abhiyan', then it should be for all children, disabled and non-disabled, instead of specialised services outside the existing structures. This requires one to look at policy, which should discourage the setting up of special institutions. And although it is believed that there will always be people who would need only vocational training or sheltered workshops, Singh questions why cannot the corporate sector take on persons with disabilities? 'After all even they have a social obligation, don't they?', she says forcefully. Singh states that one needs to examine the existing structures and see how one can work towards convergence. But till the structures open up, there is bound to be a reliance on institution-based services.

On the same subject of working with the community, Poonam Natarajan says that one of VS's methods is to set up networks with different NGOs working in different regions. Thus, when a particular NGO requests their help in the area of disability, they help them in the planning. In this way, according to Natarajan, 'we don't have to go and create the need'. Most of the work is top-down in these NGOs. Also, many of the NGOs have varied concerns and are not working specifically in the area of disability. Therefore, whatever is the NGOs' agenda, disability is also included as one of the components. Setting up self-help groups (SHGs) is one of the main activities that many of the NGOs take up. Each SHG defines its own concerns. The idea of SHGs came about because in the West the rehabilitation professionals had completely taken over the lives of the persons with disability. This made them mere passive patients who could neither do anything nor think for, and by themselves. Thus, as a mark of protest and to emphasise the need for independence in decision-making, the disabled led the move to the formation of SHGs.

Commenting on the concept of CBR, Anita Ghai raised certain crucial questions: 'The community in India is not so simple to understand. And there is really no community participation. There are no such homogeneous communities'. The major problem with the programme is that it is top-down in approach not bottom-up. For instance, when you talk of education, it is couched in terms of special education—why? It is true that some of the disabled will require special aids. Employment comes when there are basic skills. If no attention is paid to that, and only employment by itself is emphasised, then one will again remain in the charity mode. One needs to develop capabilities. Inclusion does not mean that you throw someone into the water without a tyre. Inclusion means that you will provide the tyre (assistance) that is required.

The themes and concerns discussed earlier draw attention to the fact that a welfare state concern has been absent all along with respect to the disabled in India. One of the reasons for very little being done for the disabled can be the economic factor about value attached to 'able-bodied labour'. In India, there is so much surplus labour, as well as cheap labour, that replacing the labour of a disabled person has been easy. As a result, there was no need to rehabilitate the disabled labour in order to return it to the labour market for further use. Another factor is the long-standing dominance of the charity mode of provisions for the disabled. The charity orientation overshadowed the concerns of the disabled as any other marginalised group's demands for rights.

A fuller understanding of why the disabled never came under the purview of the Indian welfare state model can be obtained from Nirja Jayal's analysis of the Indian welfare state. She argues that the United

Kingdom and other countries of the industrialised world recovering from the economic and personnel havoc created by the Second World War required government assistance and benefits to recover the economy and provide livelihood to the categories of people most affected. Similarly, in India given the social, economic and political situation and the numerous human problems resulting from the partition of the country and in the mainly agriculture-based economy, there was an increased demand requiring urgent attention in the necessity of types, quality, quantity and level of services determined by the availability of resources.

However, the implementation of the welfare state model in India seems from the outset to have been overburdened with contradiction and frustrations. According to Jayal (1994, 18–26), in the twin context of challenges to the welfare state in the West, and the policies of economic reform initiated in India, it is widely believed that the Indian state is reneging on its welfare promises, and thereby compromising its fundamental defining ideals.

In re-examining whether India is, or ever was, a welfare state in the sense in which Western political theory and practice define it, Jayal argues that indeed it is true that India does not fulfil many of the definitional criteria associated with the welfare states of the West. In the world of its origins, the institution of the welfare state was historically inspired by the intention to provide a corrective mechanism, compensating for market-generated inequalities; in India, according to Jayal, the state's assumption of welfare tasks—however narrowly defined—paralleled the embarkation on a state-directed and essentially capitalist path of development. Thus, the Indian state can be characterised as an interventionist and developmentalist state, with only a limited welfarist orientation.

In the Indian context, the arguments for the rolling back of the state have in recent times generally echoed a variant of the efficiency argument. The critique of the public sector has primarily targeted its inefficiency and wastefulness. It is argued that not only do the benefits of welfare schemes not reach their intended beneficiaries, but also that the concern for social justice has itself led to faulty economic and planning policies. Jayal also points out that the moral aspect of the neoliberal critique of the welfare state in the West has been altogether absent in the Indian context. She argues that rights' claims have not been a component of the neoliberal agenda in India, not least because rights have never been central to the philosophy of welfare that underpins the welfarist initiatives of the Indian state. Since welfare is not expressed in terms of rights, its abandonment could arguably be a relatively simple matter. A right that has never been *conferred* is self-evidently difficult to claim or defend. Thus, the question of rights is altogether external to the debate, not only in the form of libertarian notion of rights, strictly ruling out state interventionism, but also in the possible form of a radical notion of social rights in which claims to welfare may conceivably be grounded.

It is suggested that the Indian state may be more appropriately characterised as an interventionist rather than a welfare state. Interventionism can subsume a welfarist orientation. The primary purpose of interventionism and its inspiring and guiding force was developmentalist. This was not a state that self-consciously and deliberately took on the responsibility of providing for its citizens, in clearly defined areas which bore some relationship to the idea of needs, especially basic needs. Instead the paramount concern of the post-colonial Indian state was the project of modernisation. The developmental initiatives of the state were largely directed to the industrial sector. In the strategy of development planning, the economic component of development was privileged over its social and political aspects. The gradualist approach to democratic social transformation necessitated the acceptance of structural inequalities.

There are two relevant grounds for a philosophy of welfare: a needs-based conception of justice and a theory of rights and obligations. In terms of the theoretical distinction, the philosophy of welfare adopted by the Indian state has two notable aspects: the first is that of the rights enshrined in the Fundamental Rights given in the Constitution, whereas welfare rights are in the form of non-justiciable

Directive Principles of State Policy. This has resulted in a disjuncture between liberty rights and welfare rights in the Constitution. Second, the Indian state adheres to a needs-based conception of justice in theory, but in practice follows a philosophy of welfare manifestly based in ideas of charity and benevolence. The idea of a *right to welfare* is precluded. Hence, the question of welfare is not subject to political negotiation.

According to Ali Baquer (1994, 21), the concept of a benevolent, all-embracing and all-providing welfare state has undergone substantial change. This is not only in India but also in the most advanced countries where resources are not desperately scarce and population is 'not multiplying at an alarming rate outstripping all programmes aimed at expediting social change', as he puts it. Governments in various countries unable to maintain an acceptable standard began to dismantle the myth that a welfare state was created as perfect, flawless and the ultimate answer to the needs of all people in an attempt to promote social justice, human dignity and equality. Within five decades of its conception and the inception of the welfare state, its boundaries have got blurred, according to Baquer (1994, 21). From the ideology of the state being the only provider of services, the shift has been towards the values of market and commercial concepts of cost-effectiveness.

The shift away from the state as provider of services has been accompanied by the advocacy of NGO-based service delivery and more recently by the CBR paradigm. An in-depth examination of a CBR programme in India may be useful at this point, and one such example of the development and evaluation of the CBR project has been provided by Ajit Dalal (1998, 1–5). According to Dalal, probably in the history of social services, no other concept has become as popular in such a short time as CBR. It began as an international movement with the growing realisation that institution-based services require higher costs and do not integrate people with disability into society. CBR was regarded as a new approach in which families and communities are given the responsibility for the welfare of their members with disabilities. The success of CBR lies in encouraging people with disability, their families and the local community to join the programme.

According to Dalal (1998, 1–5), in developing countries like India, the prevalence of disability, particularly polio and blindness, is at least four times more among those who are below the poverty line than those above it are. The success of preventive and rehabilitative measures is largely dependent on the success of community development programmes. In this context, improving the quality of life of people with disabilities and their families would also benefit a large disadvantaged section of society. The emerging view today is that CBR programmes need to draw their resources from existing community development programmes and should get integrated with them.

It was with this ideological framework within which the Sirathu CBR Project took shape. Sirathu tehsil consists of 5 villages and is about 70 km from Allahabad city. It is one of the most backward regions of the Allahabad district. Barring a few high caste families, most of the inhabitants belong to lower caste, are illiterate and work as agricultural labourers.

Two features of the region worth noting were the high degree of caste consciousness among the two groups who do not trust each other and compete for scarce resources. The other feature is the prevailing ethos of dependency on external agencies for rehabilitation. The culture of dependency has been built up over the last 40 to 45 years and is sustained by the practice of 'welfare' camps. In these camps, aids and appliances are distributed free of cost by government and non-government agencies. Self-reliance is least appealing in this set-up and any initiative to mobilise local resources is viewed with scepticism.

Ajit Dalal and others were part of a project, which was looking at the setting up, working and evaluation of CBR projects across South Asia. The Sirathu Project was part of that study. The Sirathu Project did achieve moderate success despite many constraints and compulsions. The project also threw up questions for the CBR approach. First, it is presumptuous to imagine that village communities are cohesive and motivated. In reality, they are often faction-ridden with different interest groups operating at cross purposes. CBR programmes are highly vulnerable to local influences. Experience indicates that rehabilitation programmes succeed where local leadership is strong and has a high moral standing. Second, a major challenge for a CBR programme is to bring about attitudinal change. In a culture where suffering is accepted as karma, where people below subsistence levels have learned to reconcile themselves to their helplessness, any talk of CBR is a distant dream. According to Dalal (1998, 1–5), one has to give serious consideration to see how CBR can work in a community which is oppressed and exploited for centuries. The rehabilitation work in such a situation cannot be divorced from the larger concerns of socio-economic development. Third, in a resource-starved underdeveloped village, only a low-cost CBR is viable. The dictum is self-sustenance rather than self-reliance. According to Dalal (1998, 1–5), 'It is tragic that the many government schemes for disabled people remain out of reach for those who require them. Success of any community effort is to be assessed in terms of revival of these defunct schemes. For this, the communities should be motivated to work as a pressure group to claim benefits for their disabled members and their families'.

The aforementioned discussion about CBR and the example of a CBR project in a backward village in India has brought to light some of logistical difficulties with the CBR approach. However, one thing that the discussion did not highlight is the role of the family, especially the mother/woman who would be doing most of the looking after of the disabled person under CBR, and we need to bear in mind the features of the gender biases in the ideologies of caring that was discussed in Chapter 2.

Summing up, a survey of the policies, the legislative interventions and the interviews with professionals and disability activists suggests that the state has failed to create a coherent agenda for disabled people in terms of the implementation of the legal frame of obligation and the institutional means by which needs can be translated into practical claims. According to Harriss-White (1999, 153), there has also been a consistent trend of real decline in the resources allotted to alleviating disabilities, to which a miniscule fraction of those needing support actually gain access. The state also fails to regulate both the private sector and NGOs with any consistency. Hence, the inevitable impact on state underfunding and of the dispersed and joint responsibilities of state and a variety of NGOs with limited, self-defined briefs has been made public in a series of case studies of the arbitrary sterilisation of mentally retarded girls committed by courts to a segregated institution in Maharashtra; in a situation of inadequate, undertrained and under-remunerated staffing, water shortages, underfeeding and insanitary conditions, sexual harassment, a recourse to arbitrary and technically illegal surgical interventions was used as a technical solution to social problems (P. Bidwai in Harriss-White 1999, 152).

Thus, according to Harriss-White (1999, 152–153), 'in setting its current welfare priorities, the state has ducked responsibility for disabled people and is currently unwilling, rather than unable, to substitute for the market or the various charitable institutions proxying for the "community"'. Given the wider framework of the political economy in which the state is retreating from its earlier welfarist obligations, which may not have ever been put into practice but were recognised at least at the conceptual level, the debate on disability tends to be confined to a state versus NGO, and an institutional versus CBR paradigm. However, the issue being missed out is that from the point of view of the disabled, the state and the NGOs, or institutions and CBR, are not contradictory but complementary to each other. The stability of state resources, the framework of rights and the capacity to reach widely into the countryside which only the state has, is a necessary component of any disability programme even when the NGOs are a part of the service delivery system and CBR facilitates the incorporation of the disabled into their communities.

The Welfare State as Paternalistic Caregiver

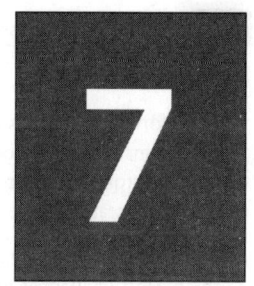

While campaigning for elections in 2010 in the United Kingdom, David Cameron, who himself had a child with CP, made a fervent plea for the state providing care to the disabled. With great eloquence he said:

> My son Ivan was born with a profound disability, and my experience of looking after him has changed the way I see a lot of things—not just as a father, but as a politician, too. Samantha and I went on a steep learning curve. From that I learned five big lessons that have had a direct impact on what my party wants to do in government for those with disabilities and their families.
>
> The first lesson I learned was the importance of early intervention and help. The day you find out your child has a disability you're not just deeply shocked, worried and upset—you're also incredibly confused.
>
> The second lesson was that life for parents of a child with disability is complicated enough without having to jump through hundreds of government hoops. After the initial shock of diagnosis you're plunged into a world of bureaucratic pain.
>
> The third lesson is that we've got to make it easier for parents to get the right education for children with disabilities. So many parents get stuck on a merry-go-round of assessments, appeals and tribunals to get a statement of special needs and the extra help their child needs.
>
> Something else that many parents have to fight tooth and nail for is a place in a special school. Following the gospel of inclusion, the Government has closed dozens of special schools down in the last decade. Inclusion is

great for some, but it's often the case that putting a child with disability in a mainstream classroom is a square peg-round-hole situation. So we're going to stop the closure of special schools and give parents more information and greater choice.

The fourth lesson is that like all other carers, parents need a break. One of the biggest challenges when your child is severely disabled is finding time to do normal family stuff—playing in the park with your other children, doing the weekly shop, mum and dad going out for a meal.

Respite made a massive difference to my family. Knowing that Ivan was with people who knew him, who would love and look after him gave us a huge wave of relief. Backing respite means backing the voluntary sector, giving parents and carers greater choice over the respite that suits them and looking at all ways of making sure there's a clear entitlement to respite.

The fifth and final lesson I'm going to share is this. The very painful thing about disability—whether your own or your loved one's—is the feeling that the situation is out of your control. When the system that surrounds you is very top-down, very bureaucratic, very inhuman, that can only increase your feelings of helplessness. So a really big difference we can make is to put more power and control right into the hands of parents, carers or those with disabilities through personal budgets and direct payments. That means that instead of giving a little bit of money from health, from education, from children's services, we say to people: 'Here is the total budget for you or your child, you choose how it's broken down'. And instead of insisting on separate, bureaucratic bank accounts for that money, it is right people should be paid directly if they choose. This is the support, trust and respect that parents of those with disabilities deserve.

Because we can never forget what an amazing job they do. Just consider what it would mean if the army of parents and carers in this country gave up, packed up, said they couldn't cope any more. The financial cost of looking after those children would be immense—and the emotional cost doesn't bear thinking about. We need to recognise that by staying strong and holding their families together, these parents are doing a great, unsung service to our society. (Cameron 2009)

But in January 2011, after Cameron had been elected, a news item reported:

> David Cameron was yet to write to a mother who may have to put her severely disabled daughter into care.

Riven Vincent, from Bristol, told the online forum Mumsnet that she could no longer cope with the day-to-day care of Celyn, six, who is blind, quadriplegic and has cerebral palsy and epilepsy.

In her message, she wrote that her local authority, South Gloucestershire Council, had refused to provide her with extra respite support to help with her daughter's care.

She wrote: 'Have asked [social services] to take [my daughter] into care. We get six hours respite a week. They have refused a link family. They have refused extra respite. I can't cope'. (Community Care 2011)

These citations graphically reveal an inconvenient truth about an erstwhile welfare state which is systematically turning its back on its promise of support. At the same time, the passages also reveal that lifelong caregiving and its consequences are at the heart of the experience of families which have children with CP, and the stress can be unbearable without external support from the state. In a fundamental sense then the state is/or can be the paternalistic caregiver that can reduce the stress levels and improve the quality of life for both the child with special needs and the parents who have the primary responsibility of providing care. It is necessary, therefore, to examine the history and workings of the 'welfare' state and the manner in which the state has responded to the needs of its citizens, especially those located at the margins of society—the underprivileged, the elderly and the disabled, historically over time, and in its contemporary settings.

Concern about disability has a long history, which has been reflected in the economy, the level of technology, class interests and ideology of the times. Hence, in this context, it is important to understand the development of the welfare state and the various social welfare policies regarding disability and rehabilitation the world over.

The term welfare is popularly associated with some form of economic or non-economic benefits to persons who need support, which they are not able to otherwise secure for themselves. The provider of such support can be a governmental body, religious body, occupational guild and non-governmental or voluntary organisation.

However, in the context of a welfare policy, it is the role of the government that comes into prominence. Many theorists and social analysts have attempted to formulate the kind of welfare policy that should be adopted by the state. Chatterjee (1997) has cited Hill and noted that it is not possible to separate social policy from economic policy because both involve the redistribution of income. Marshall in Chatterjee (1997) called welfare policy 'the policy of governments with regard to action having a direct impact on the welfare of citizens by providing them with services or income'. Titmuss in Chatterjee (1997) defined welfare policy as 'provisions by collectivities' to deal with various 'states of dependency'. Various reasons have been given for the context of the emergence of the welfare state; for example, Goodin suggested in Chatterjee (1997) that the welfare state is set in the context of the market economy and is an attempt to modify the market forces in various limited respects. Its function, however, is not to supplant the market altogether. Esping-Andersen in Chatterjee (1997) stated that the development of the welfare state can be understood from three dimensions: (a) the roles of the state and the market in making allocations, (b) the impact of the welfare state on society's hierarchies and (c) the process by which certain allocations become entitlements. Thus, variations in social welfare policies are seen as guided by variations in the values and ideologies of given societies, variations in the techno-economic bases and market fluctuations within and around given societies, and also that social welfare policies are a camouflage for inherent class and interest group conflicts in society. Thus, there are different social and economic models of welfare; Titmuss has identified welfare as a residual burden, as complementarity and as an instrument of equality.

The development of the 'Welfare State' is seen in a historical perspective as a part of a broad, ascending path of social betterment provided for the working classes since the 19th century. However, state participation in the regulation or policies for the provision of welfare to the people has a longer history. Leichter (1979, 15–27) has identified three historical periods in the origins and evolution of state activity in welfare. The first begins with the emergence of the modern nation-state in the 16th century up to the latter part of the 18th century in Europe and parts of Asia. During this period, the centralised, positive state first appeared. Thus, the range and effectiveness of the state activity was in providing defence and maintaining internal order; public finance; social and economic regulatory policy; and social welfare. Paternalism was the concept that led to the development of state-supported welfare or poor relief programmes. By the 17th century, virtually every European state had some sort of centrally established public welfare programme. One of the first was the Grand Bureau des Pauvres established in France in 1550; the Elizabethan Poor Law, passed in 1601; a Russian system of state-operated welfare established during the reign of Peter the Great (1682–1725); and the Prussian system of poor relief that evolved various edicts between 1596 and 1703. Although there was considerable variation in control and operation among the programmes, nevertheless there were certain common elements in the features then and some have links with the modern concept and operation of welfare systems. One feature was that the motivation behind early welfare systems was not exclusively paternalistic or religious. In many instances, poor relief was an exercise of the state's police power. Throughout the 16th to 18th centuries, in Europe and elsewhere, landless peasants, persons uprooted by war and returning and unemployed soldiers resorted to vagrancy, begging, stealing and extortion to support themselves. Hence, the 'welfare' policies were another way of dealing with the problems of maintaining law and order.

Early health welfare policies were related to the doctrine of mercantilism, the reasoning being that the power and wealth of the state depended on a healthy and vigorous, large population.

Another common feature was the legal distinction between categories or types of needy people. The primary distinction was between those who were legitimately poor (e.g., the aged, insane, blind or otherwise physically handicapped) and the able-bodied 'scoundrels', 'rogues' and professional beggars. Each category of persons was treated differently: for example, institutional relief (alms houses) were for the 'deserving' poor; workhouses for the able-bodied poor who were willing to work; and punishment for the able-bodied unwilling to work. From the very beginning, poor relief was deemed as justified only in case of severe disability.

A third common feature was the assumption that each locality should be held responsible for its own poor and needy. Although the laws were centrally promulgated, they were to be financed and administered by local authorities.

A final common feature of these welfare programmes was that the acceptance of public relief carried with it considerable social stigma, marking the recipient as socially inferior. There were, at times, not only social but also legal sanctions imposed on those who had to turn to public welfare assistance.

The second period, beginning in some nations early in the 19th century, was that of the Industrial Revolution in much of Western Europe. This period was characterised in some nations by a more limited concept of the role the state should perform. The set of ideas that supported the view of the limited state was summarised by the phrase 'laissez-faire'. These ideas were first advocated by the English and French philosophers and economists during the late 18th and early 19th centuries. Laissez-faire emphasised natural laws and individual rights of the propertied, rejected government paternalism and intervention and, therefore, appeared better suited to the new economic order. Although never adopted as the only guide for formulating public policy, it did have a profound impact in Europe, the US and the colonies of Asia and Africa. But as industrialisation proceeded in the more advanced nations, it brought with it a changing social, economic and political environment. And the laissez-faire began to appear inadequate in the face of the social and political consequences of industrialisation.

The third period beginning roughly in the latter part of the 19th century was marked by the adverse consequences of the shift from a primarily agrarian to a primarily industrial economic base; these changes produced, and continue to produce, extraordinary societal dislocations and profound social and economic changes. During the course of the 19th century, it became clear to many that the social and economic dislocations and human misery spawned by industrialisation required remedial action beyond that which was provided by private charities, and that state intervention was needed. A more receptive environment of state involvement existed in Germany, Austria and Russia where paternalism persisted over laissez-faire. However, in England, France and the US, where laissez-faire had its strongest advocates, the doctrine was losing support in favour of a more activist and positive concept of state to provide protection against the evils and insecurities of industrialisation. The documentation of extreme levels of exploitation by humanist reformers helped to disseminate awareness about the consequences of industrialisation and created the climate for reconceptualising the role of the state and its responsibilities towards its people.

One of the most significant shifts that occurred was from the concept of poor law relief to the idea of social insurance. As industrialisation and socio-economic insecurity advanced, the increasingly large, vocal and educated urban working class began organising, demanding and receiving greater political power. With the end of the extended family system, the needs of the urban worker for protection from the insecurities associated with loss of wages owing to industrial injuries, disability, illness, unemployment and old age increased resulting in the demand for social security.

The first modern and comprehensive social security programme was developed during the 1880s. Chancellor Otto von Bismarck introduced laws for sickness insurance (1883), accident insurance (1884) and invalidity and old-age insurance (1889; Leichter 1979, 110). One of the factors in Bismarck's radical social programme was the Prussian tradition of the paternalistic state and its concern for the needy. Shortly after the introduction of social insurance programmes in Germany, several nations followed such as Austria, Czechoslovakia (injury insurance, 1887; sickness insurance, 1888; old-age disability insurance, 1906), Denmark (between 1897 and 1896), Italy (between

1898 and 1919) and Great Britain (between 1897 and 1911). By the second decade of the 20th century, most advanced nations in the world had a relatively comprehensive social insurance programme. The major exception was the US, which did not have a job-related illness or injury insurance programme until 1908, and an old age, disability and survivor's insurance programme was set up only in 1935 as part of the New Deal in response to the social distress following the collapse of the economy in 1929.

According to Vicente Navarro (1999, 1–50), the most important causes of the evolution of the funding and organisation of the welfare state are political. Although the basis for establishing the welfare state preceded the Second World War, its full development took place after the war, in the golden age of capitalism. This development varied with the political tradition that became dominant in each country. Of these political traditions, four were particularly important: the Social Democratic, the Christian Democratic, the Fascist and the Liberal.

Social democratic public policies were for the most part developed in the northern European countries of Sweden, Norway, Denmark and Finland and also in Austria. In these countries, the labour movement had two instruments to defend its interests: the unions and the social democratic parties. The objective was to expand political and social rights of the entire population through solidarity and universalisation of such rights. In order to achieve universality, the aim was to achieve full employment and to establish a welfare state that protected citizens throughout their life cycle and through redistributive policies to reduce social inequalities created by the market. The achievement of full employment required the active participation of both men and women in the labour force. Hence, the state had to provide a series of services to the families and particularly to women to enable women to enter paid employment. The extensive welfare services included health care, education and social services to the vulnerable populations such as the children, the elderly and the disabled.

The Christian Democratic countries include Belgium, Germany and the Netherlands. In these countries, the family and the life cycle have defined the welfare state. The male was the head of the family, the breadwinner responsible for the family's economic stability, which depended on his wages and pension. The wife took care of elders and children. Hence, the key economic element, the standard of living and welfare of the family was based on the salary and pension of the male member working in the labour force. The public policies regarding pensions and other benefits for workers depended on their status within the hierarchy in the production process and in society. The women in these countries worked at home—even in the 1980s only 46 per cent of women worked in the labour market (compared with 65 per cent in the social democratic countries). Since the women worked at home, looking after the dependents, the scenario resulted in the poor development or absence of childcare services or domiciliary home care services for the elderly and the disabled. The underdevelopment of the social services created a burden for the families, especially for women. According to Navarro, characteristic of the Christian Democratic public policies is that the responsibilities of care are assigned to different agents of civil society. Hence, voluntarism is the key means of calling on people's altruism and compassion. Navarro considers it important to clarify that it is profoundly wrong to try to replace the welfare state by voluntarism and a call for family responsibility. The welfare state and welfare society should be complementary rather than mutually exclusive.

The welfare states in southern European countries such as Spain, Greece and Portugal have been heavily influenced by long periods of dictatorship. These countries had poorly developed social services. A characteristic that these countries share with the Christian Democratic countries is their emphasis on the family and on women as being responsible for the care of children and the elderly.

The public policies of the liberal countries including those that have never been governed by social democratic parties, for example, Canada and the US and those governed by such parties for a long period, for example, Great Britain, are residual and assistential. Such welfare state policies provide services and benefits based on proven financial need (tested) rather than as a matter of citizen or worker's rights. There are exceptions such as the universal health services in Canada and Britain. The liberal model assigns welfare responsibilities to the private sector, once the minimums are guaranteed by the state.

This survey of the different approaches to welfare indicates that in sum welfare is not an adjunct to the economy but a part of the economy and impacts the experience of health, and disability, adding to reducing the quantum of suffering for those at the bottom end of society.

REHABILITATION POLICIES

Rehabilitation is a component of the health care system, which develops after full attention has been given to acute care and reduction of mortality. General health policies and systems typically precede rehabilitation. The diseases and health conditions which adversely affect health status also produce the disability that requires rehabilitation. In order to plan a national rehabilitation policy, it is important to define disability. The manner in which the state defines its relationship to 'welfare' crucially determines the rehabilitation policies it will adopt towards its vulnerable sections, particularly the 'disabled'.

Even before a more generalised notion of welfare came to be significant, frequently national and local communities had acted to protect those citizens judged to be most valuable for the survival of a particular institution. The US began providing disability benefits for merchant seamen in 1798 at a time when control of the sea lanes and maintenance of a strong fleet was critical to the security and commerce of the country. Similarly, benefits for soldiers were provided during war times, and compensation and aid was provided to railroad workers during the 19th century to maintain a skilled labour force necessary for the industrial revolution. Individual social positions were principally dependent upon occupational attainment, based on the value of labour expressed in earnings and prestige. Disability benefits, in turn, generally were determined by an individual's relative position in the labour force and the likelihood of his return to work after rehabilitation. According to Albrecht and Levy (Albrecht 1981, 11), these actions reflect the political economy and ruling class interests as well as values of those in power.

Anne Crichton has examined policy development of rehabilitation policies in Britain, Canada and Australia for they share the same language and culture (Albrecht 1981, 157–180). Their approach to solving social problems is similar in terms of their thought processes; ideologies and social structures have common historical origins. Yet differences in social policies have emerged because of the different resources at their disposal and different environmental and social pressures. Hence, the words 'policy' and 'rehabilitation' tend to be defined differently by all who choose to use them.

Taking a historical approach to the development of rehabilitation policy for the disabled, Crichton has analysed what the three countries deemed to be 'deserving' groups for state-mediated schemes for injured/diseased workmen and war veterans, the blind, the crippled, the totally disabled and the elderly.

In Britain, with the breakup of the Poor Law and the attempt at post-war reconstruction, there was a review of the condition of the British people and their needs for social services. The 'welfare state' was chosen as the solution to deal with problems of improving social organisation. The 'welfare state' was to provide not only cash when necessary but services in kind to ensure 'equality of opportunity' and 'equality of condition' for all citizens from 'the cradle to the grave'.

Beveridge's classification of groups to be considered for social security coverage revealed that 'employability' was basic to his thinking. And for those who were unable to be employed there would be social assistance. According to Crichton, it was necessary, however, to make an exception of the disabled and to develop special provisions for them in addition to the general welfare state services because of their problems in getting work. In addition to having open access to the general welfare state provisions, Disablement Resettlement Officers were made responsible for assessing and placing registered persons with disability in open or sheltered employment. Employers were obliged to take a fixed percentage of workers with disability and some jobs were to be kept for persons with disability (Albrecht 1981, 157–180).

In Canada, during the post-war reconstruction, Beveridge's research assistant Marsh prepared a report as cited in Crichton (1981, 164). The two main outcomes of the report were that the federal government should (a) provide pensions to identified groups of individuals in need of income maintenance and (b) to provide matching grants to provincial governments of specified social programmes.

The Canadian Pension Plan of 1965 subsumed the specific income maintenance programmes developed in the early 1950s for the blind, the totally disabled and crippled children into a general minimum income programme for designated groups. In 1966, the Canada Assistance Plan was introduced. This provided matching grants for institutional programmes for groups in special need and enabled many people with disability to be given more care than they had had in the province's old established asylums. Gradually with such shifts in the care, structure, attitudes to stigmatisation started changing towards the retarded, the elderly and others who had been put in residential care earlier. The public health service was closely linked with educational provision for the children with disability who needed support, whether in special schools or classes, or who had to be provided with special help in ordinary classrooms or at home. For the support of the persons with disability who had passed beyond the school's system, an act to facilitate the vocational rehabilitation of persons with disability was passed in 1961.

The Australian commitment to the 'welfare state' was much more cautious than that of the other two countries. The federal government had an income maintenance scheme in the Invalid and Old-age Pensions Act 1941.

According to Crichton (1981, 157–180), while the British 'welfare state' attempted to reconcile universalistic approaches to support through income maintenance for all citizens with particularistic approaches to support through the national health service (NHS) and personal social services, other governments devised different schemes. Canada accepted the British principles at the federal level. The Australians seemed to have been less convinced that the whole range of policies were necessary. This belief in selective rather than universal policies resulted in the development of special policies to support the disabled. The government became aware of the need for an improved disablement rehabilitation service for vocational retraining because at the end of the Second World War more than half the men and women discharged from the armed services were medically unfit and were eligible for veteran's benefits.

While the Australians were less willing than the British or Canadians to become committed to a NHS or health insurance scheme, they had, early on, developed universal public health services within states which provided maternity and child welfare, assessment of handicaps and support for children with disabilities.

In order to move towards a more comprehensive rehabilitation policy, the disabled groups became active in demanding their human rights since the 1970s in Western democratic countries. They raised major issues about the meaning of equal citizenship, the meaning of work in society, how individual worth is assessed and how those who deviate from the norm should be identified and classified.

In the 1960s, in Britain, the severely disabled began to form visible and effective pressure groups whose activity resulted in the Chronically Sick and Disabled Persons Act, 1970. Two principles were given recognition: first the importance of providing community care for those who did not wish to be housed in institutions, and second, the need for providing higher allowances for those who were living at the subsistence level, not temporarily but for long periods of time. However, a consciousness was emerging that the 'welfare state', in its concern for general social well-being had failed many who fell through the gaps between departments of the social service delivery system. There was an awareness within the hospital system that rehabilitation was inadequate and that there were discrepancies between the needs of the elderly and the disabled for health care. For instance, New Zealand had been the forerunner of a separate and different kind of criticism of the welfare state services to the handicapped. The report of a Royal Commission on Compensation and Rehabilitation, 1967, stirred the English-speaking countries to reconsider fundamental principles underlying their policies.

In Canada, in the 1960s, the groups of the disabled embarked on a crusade to improve their image and status and to make a case for better treatment, for de-stigmatisation of the disabled and redistribution of resources. However, they had considerable difficulty in deciding courses of action because the existing structures set up to assist the disabled were so complex and the principles underlying policies to support them were unclear. In a review of programmes and policies for the disabled by the Canadian Department of National Health and Welfare (1971), it was shown that despite improvements in general provision of services introduced in the 1960s, particularistic services were not well developed.

In Australia, there was a Community Health and Hospitals programme, which was a plan to begin the redistribution of resources away from high technology medicine to community care. This helped the chronically sick and disabled in the community.

An analysis of the policies in the three countries and their differing response to pressures indicates that while Britain was more concerned about equalisation policies because it is well aware that privilege is still entrenched, Canada and Australia are perceived to be countries where there is greater equality of citizenship. The dominant ideology of the three countries of a Western liberal democratic faith was modified to a different extent in each of the countries. The challenge to resource development as the best solution to improvement of the citizenship rights came from the socialists, who were concerned because unrestricted liberalism seemed to be a denial of equality and fraternity and because it created so many casualties along the way. Thus, the balancing of utilitarian and humanitarian policies became the challenge to liberal democratic societies. According to Crichton, Beveridge thought he had found a solution in the 'welfare state' concept, but critics of this concept such as Wilding and George, in Crichton (1981, 176) stated that rather than correcting, it compounds injustice because of its failures in dealing with the issue of fairer redistribution of resources.

All the three 'welfare state' approaches were utilitarian in the liberal democratic tradition as their services for the disabled make clear. These were all directed to low-level income maintenance for invalids and vocational rehabilitation. Australia did not retreat far from the concept of 'residual welfare' (individual responsibility) while Britain, and to a lesser extent Canada, showed some concern for those who were trapped in an unfair economic system. In the early days of the welfare state, Britain campaigned strongly for de-stigmatisation of the disabled, though the attempts at removal of discrimination were not successful. However, attitude changes in Canada and Australia were more difficult and the disabled continued to be stigmatised along with deviant groups.

Walker and Townsend have summarised in Crichton (1981, 179) the themes that had been emerging in public discussion during the 1960s and early 1970s: 'There was the growing desire on the part of the disabled for self-determination and access to jobs and ordinary roles in society.' There was the demand of women for parity in treatment with men, for example in calling attention to the rights of disabled women. Most of all, there was reaction from many sources of opinion against the fragmentation and inequality in the treatment of disabled people implied by dividing them according to type or cause of disability.

Hall et al. have discussed in Crichton (1981, 179), how issues make their way into the system and become policies. One important feature of success is to get attached to other social policies, which are popular and well supported. For example, the blind made great progress when they associated themselves with ex-servicemen. Crichton (1981, 179) feels that now that the disabled have become visible as a group entitled to their human rights, others may hang on to them, but it will be necessary for them to recognise that, essentially, they are a deviant group, tolerated and made the objects of sympathy. Humanitarianism has its limits in utilitarian liberal democratic societies and even with improved recognition of the needs of the disabled, there will be hesitations in meeting these needs. It is for this reason that preventive policies are most urgently desired.

According to Gary Albrecht's (1981, 269) critical assessment of cross-national rehabilitation policies, the perceived salience of disability as a social problem, the accumulation of surplus capital and the growth of the welfare state have contributed to the development of extensive rehabilitation polices rationalised in terms of the national interest. Any thoughtful analysis of these national rehabilitation policies is sensitive to the social history and political economy of individual countries that make them unique. However, comparative policy analysis forces us to think in terms of the development of general principles and theoretical models.

In conclusion, it can be stated that there are general principles and models in the development of health service systems of a nation. Yet their utility is limited by the many intervening variables that affect health policy implementation. Hence, an understanding of cross-national rehabilitation policies is dependent upon an appreciation of the corresponding national health systems designed primarily to diagnose and treat potentially disabling conditions. Disability benefits are generally contingent on the individual's ability to perform social roles. However, with the definitions of disability expanding the scope of the rehabilitation services for the population at risk has also to be enlarged proportionately. The progressive disenchantment with the medical model of rehabilitation led to the development of the social service model of rehabilitation. Presently, the integration of the disabled into mainstream society is the main plank of the crusade. Although in most of the developed countries nutritional and communicable disease problems are solved, this is not so in the developing countries and the effects of chronic illness become increasingly apparent in both sets of countries. The problems and available solutions of industrial countries are different from those in less developed countries, therefore, different interventions are required. However, with changing political, economic and social conditions, nations will be forced to make social choices concerning the identification and treatment of disabilities.

According to Marshall, the welfare state was born into a world of austerity—of rationing, price control, coupons and rent restrictions. It was not that these restrictions on the free market were regarded as good, in themselves, and as desirable elements in the new social order (Marshall 1964, 322). But they provided a background to welfare legislation, a society committed to 'fair shares' and to distribution of income, which could be rationally justified and was not the unpredictable result of the supposedly blind forces of a competitive market in which everybody was entitled to take as much as he/she could get.

By the mid-1950s and early 1960s, the 'Austerity society' had passed away and the 'Affluent society' was taking its place. The restraints on self-enrichment and competitive consumption were removed, and sensational stories of astronomic salaries, limitless expense accounts and fabulous speculative gains in real estate and elsewhere (some of the things the Indian media has circulated in the last few years as part of the promotion of the liberalisation model) were told. Prices rose, wage demands became an annual event and inflation deprived some of the welfare benefits of their original value. It was in these circumstances that the basic principles of the welfare state came under attack. The main objectives of the attack were the principle of universality and the provision of certain services free to all.

A series of parallel developments and complementary processes were unfolding in the US. At the end of the Second World War, the US emerged as the sole hegemonic capitalist power, dominant in the economic, political and military spheres. Under the US leadership, a set of international institutions were developed to provide viable international trade. The rapid growth of world trade, the spread of MNCs and the development of international credit resulted in a close interdependence of the capitalist nations on one another—all through the centralisation of the state structure was visible.

But towards the end of the 1970s, the boom of post-war economic growth came to a halt and caused global recession. The growth in the welfare state globally came to an abrupt end in many countries. Simultaneously, the collapse of the Soviet Union and the nations of the socialist block in the late 1980s led to the reshaping of the capitalist world and a possibility to pressurise for a return to the laissez-faire liberalism by reducing state interference to a minimum. The theoretical perspective of the neoliberals gained prominence and advocated the rejection of the welfare state principle. This was the period of the neoliberals' first electoral success with the election of the Reagan and Thatcher governments in the US and Britain. Their right-wing economic policies reflected the ideological commitment to unbridled market principles, ignoring the remarkable role of state-directed economies in these countries, wherein state involvement in public health had been central to the strategy to stabilise the economies in a move to help capital growth and technological change. Thus, by the 1980s, the welfare model was being countered globally and echoed nationally. Public expenditure was cut back and within this total, social expenditure suffered the most.

However, this new wave of neoliberalism and reform strategies for health care has resulted in privatisation of health care and the commodifying of health. The main arguments for privatisation are cost-efficiency and that since individuals are rational beings, they should be allowed to make the choice that they most desire in the larger democratic interest. Due to the emphasis on state withdrawal from the welfare sector, in general, a major consequence of privatisation is that the state has also abdicated its responsibility to the welfare of its people. In the health sector, this has led to two major effects: one, that the caring of the patient has landed on the family or what is called the familialisation of health care, and second, the costs of curing have to be borne solely by the individual. The implications of such a situation for most Third-World countries, which have not achieved or ensured the basics of food, clean water, health, education and employment for all, are such that the scenario of state withdrawal will have a cumulative effect on the health of the people as shown in many studies from Latin America and sub-Saharan Africa.

Another feature of privatisation is the development of, and encouragement given to, the NGO sector. The NGOs are considered to be a far better conduit for the distribution of multilateral and bilateral aid in the area of social and economic development. The origins of the development of the NGOs may be traced back to around the 1970s. In India, NGOs emerged as a response to the larger retreat of institutional politics, and these organisations were viewed as political interventions within the mainstream.

The NGOs, as an alternate sector, were supposed to rectify state failure with their interventions and were seldom seen as a means to correct market failure. According to Alan Fowler, as cited in Zaidi (1999), the NGOs are thought to be more cost-effective in service delivery, to have greater ability to target the poor and vulnerable sections of the population, to demonstrate a capacity to develop community-based institutions, and to be better able to promote the popular participation needed for sustainability of benefits.

The major criticism of the NGO sector is that the NGOs are largely donor driven, generate patron–client relationships within an unequal power situation and enter only particular sectors. Tendler, as cited in Zaidi (1999), has provided evidence, which indicates that the NGOs function as top-down, non-participatory and uninnovative. Replicability and sustainability, two criteria that define the success of NGO projects, have also not been fulfilled in many cases. Because of their limited scope and reach, NGOs are no alternative to the state. Thus, many studies have revealed that regarding NGOs as an alternate development paradigm has been grossly exaggerated. According to Zaidi (1999), NGOs, at best, are providers of a minimal amount of 'band-aid social welfare'. The only alternative to state failure is the state itself because it is only the state which can provide continuity of services. In sum, in Third-World countries, a different form of state, based on a different equation with 'civil society', which is decentralised, delegatory and democratic, may perhaps be the only alternative to state failure itself.

CONCLUSION

The case for the market providing services is being ably presented by economists who argue that services collectively organised by the state are seen as a temporary economic phenomenon peculiar to a specific historical phase in the development of large-scale industrial societies. They were needed as social supports when the masses were poor, in times of war and when the future of capitalism was uncertain. These conditions, it is argued, are no longer prevalent and the 'welfare state' should wither away and people should resort to a self-regulating market. Private responsibility should replace public paternalism. In the area of health, the American model of health care is regarded as the most superior, efficient and cost-effective and is spreading its tentacles in both developed and developing countries. In this model, people are viewed as consumers, health is regarded as a commodity and profit maximisation is the aim. However, as we have seen the debates are narrowing down to a single model without recalling the range of options explored by states and societies in the past. A unipolar economic world is being accompanied by the offer of a single ideology—that of the market. The question that confronts us is: Will the experience of widespread social distress, that such a society is bound to generate, lead to another or a revised phase of a welfare state?

Conclusion
The Moral and Political Economy of Disability and Suffering

ETHICAL ISSUES AND DILEMMAS—ABORTION, NEW REPRODUCTIVE TECHNOLOGIES AND EUTHANASIA

In the course of my research work, ethical issues and dilemmas faced by my interviewees and for us as a society kept crossing my path, whether it was during the interviews, discussions with people, or in the form of sensational news reports. These ethical issues and dilemmas arose particularly in the context of new reproductive technologies, abortion and euthanasia.

Historically, induced abortions have been a source of debate and controversy. In these debates, views are divided amongst those who are pro-choice (in favour of legal abortion) and those who are pro-life (against legal abortion). The spillover of this controversy is particularly highlighted in the case of disability: The central dilemma in this debate is the foetus' right to life and the woman's right to control her body. The dilemma reaches a climax when the context is selective abortion—that is abortion based on the fact that the baby to be born will be disabled. In India, selective abortion is also done on the basis of the sex of the foetus, that is, it is the female foetuses that are often aborted even when the child is going to be 'normal'.

One argument given is that since women face the most profound impact of bearing a child with disability, they should be the sole decision-makers to either continue or terminate pregnancy. However, this is viewed as a precedent to 'eliminate' the 'unfit' in the garb of the right of a woman over her body, and by implication over the way her life will unfold. The most frequently given reasons for wanting to prevent the birth of foetuses with disabilities are to avoid the inevitable negative consequences in the following areas: economic impact on families; economic impact on society; disruption of families; quality of life of the person with a disability; and notions of 'perfection'. Another medical reasoning is that foetuses with disabilities that have little chance of surviving either in the womb or soon after birth, or those that might cause harm to the mother in some way in-utero, must be aborted.

While the debate on abortion continues unabated, many of the mothers that I spoke to had quite openly stated that if they knew that their child was going to be disabled they would not have had the child. They explained that taking recourse to such an option would have been necessitated because of the fact that the 'world is at present too tough for such people to live their life completely'. One mother who had a child with severe CP, after five miscarriages, felt it would have been better that the son had not been born, or had died at birth. At least, she said, he would not have led such a miserable life.

Mothers with two children with CP especially felt that had they known the second would also be disabled, they would definitely not have brought him/her into the world, no matter how unethical it may be to think about abortion. They said their experience of how difficult it is for persons with disability, particularly in India, makes them think that they would not like them to be subjected to a life of 'torture'. They understand that even those persons who have a severe form of disability have rights, but felt that nevertheless 'they too deserve a life of dignity', not one of stigma and apathy, which is what they experience at present.

With the advent and rapid advances in prenatal screening and diagnosis, ultrasonography and amniocentesis, in particular, have been used to assess various types of disabilities and birth defects. This has been principally so in those with a genetic origin such as Down's syndrome. These methods have made extensive inroads into the medical system in India and are creating havoc via their use for foetal sex-determination, and subsequent abortion of the female foetus. They are also being used to identify disability, although I did not come across a mother who had used the new technology to abort a foetus identified as disabled. However, mothers spoke of not having access to such technology before their children were born. For instance, one mother felt that had she known from the ultrasound or tests that there was a problem with the child before it was born, she would have definitely gone in for an abortion. She had already seen the amount of trouble her sister-in-law had experienced looking after a disabled hydrocephalic daughter.

In the course of my research work, the Niketa Mehta case made headlines in the media. Her case also set up a national debate on the issue of right to abortion versus the right to life. While abortion is legal in India, it is time bound: Only a foetus of 20 weeks or lower age can be aborted on any ground. However, some disabling conditions are revealed only after 20 weeks, in which case legally an induced abortion becomes punishable. In Niketa Mehta's case, the discovery of the 'disabling' condition of the foetus was detected beyond 20 weeks and, thus, her demand for a late term abortion was turned down by the court. The central argument of the Niketa Mehta case was the family's contention that they would not be able to afford the lifelong care of a child with disability (in this case a lifelong heart condition). Frustrated by the court's denial, the parents were widely believed to have had an induced abortion which was passed off as a miscarriage. Regardless of what the facts of the situation might have been, the debate around the aborting of an 'abnormal' child died down, at least for a while.

The science of new or assisted reproductive technologies (ART: artificial insemination by donor, superovulation, in-vitro fertilisation, embryo flushing and transfer, surrogate motherhood and sex predetermination) have been hailed as miraculous triumphs providing hope to infertile parents. They have enabled many people in the world to have biological children who otherwise would not have been able to. These people include infertile women and men; single women and men; and lesbian, gay and transgender couples who were enabled to form genetically related families. These new technologies have transformed the way reproduction is viewed. While they have created new and hopeful possibilities, there is also a need for attention to be paid to issues of health, ethics, law and policy.

One of the most promising of such genetic technologies, which potentially could be used to cure any congenital disability, is genetic therapy. If the occurrence of a particular gene mutation causes a genetic disease, gene therapy may be able to repair or replace that gene with a 'normal' one. This is known as germ-line genetic engineering. This involves changing the genetics in the reproductive cells of the subject, so that the children the subject might have after the procedure do not inherit undesirable genetic traits.

While genetic engineering is currently still more science fiction than fact, recent strides in genetic technologies remind us that it is just a matter of time before the fiction becomes reality. Prenatal genetic tests already allow identifying many of the prospective child's genetic traits. Parents conceiving through in-vitro fertilisation already have some opportunities to 'choose' their child's biological characteristics by choosing which fertilised eggs are transplanted and which are not based on the results of genetic testing.

The disability scholar Shakespeare (2003) has cautioned the implications of such strides in science. He suggested that what genetic traits we ultimately select in reproductive decision-making, or target for genetic enhancement, reflects the characteristics that we value as individuals and as a society. Often traits such as athleticism and high intelligence are considered to have 'unarguably positive value', even though they show no correlation with a higher quality of life for the individual. What they do provide is an advantage in obtaining what present-day societies across the world have determined to be the parameters of achievement for our children—excellence in sports and academics.

Other characteristics, more unarguable in their benefit to the individual (such as increased resistance to disease), or arguably more beneficial to society (such as altruism), receive significantly less attention and are likely to be undervalued. Offering another example, it has been noted that there is some correlation between some mental instabilities and artistic achievement. However, will parents select their child to be the next Van Gogh if it means the child will have mental health issues as well as artistic ability? (Shakespeare 2003). This also raises concerns about genetics with a far greater basis in history: eugenics. According to Guterman (2003), it is unlikely that eugenics will re-emerge in the same form as in the past (e.g., in laws providing for mandatory sterilisation). Still, the persistence of many of the beliefs and attitudes that historically supported eugenic policies suggest that concerns about what has been termed 'elective eugenics' (the coerced aborting of foetuses with a high risk of disability) should be taken seriously.

Thus, in India the ART have enabled many to fulfil their dreams of having a biological child despite the fact that it is a very expensive process and can affect the health of women. However, there are many ethical issues surrounding the usage of ART, especially in the Indian context. This is because the laws regarding both abortion as well as ART are not well worked out to protect the stakeholders involved. In fact, in India, abortion on account of foetal abnormality is legal while sex-selective abortion is punishable by law.

According to Ghai and Johri, although technological developments enhance the sense of choice, in reality, they tend to push decisions towards a predictable socially desirable trend. In contemporary India, the technology used to prenatally determine foetal characteristics has disadvantaged both girls and the disabled. A report on ART by Sama Resource Group for Women and Health (2006) states that it is difficult to distinguish between latent choice and social choice shaped by family, market and other agents. Unless we draw this line, there is no limit to theoretical choice, and everything including sex selection can be justified in the language of choice. What society does is to promote one variety of choice while silencing the range of options.

Closely related to the issue of abortion and ART is the issue of, and dilemma involved in, euthanasia. For instance, in the case of Mira Parikh, tests in weeks 26, 28 and 30 revealed that Parikh's baby had a fistula between the food pipe and windpipe. The tests additionally revealed that the left leg was shorter than the right one, and that there was hydrocephaly or water in the brain. Parikh wanted to abort a baby that would be born mentally retarded, but the law would not permit it. At 34 weeks, Parikh went into premature labour. The newborn boy needed intensive care but Mira chose the general ward. The fistula meant that when he suckled, milk entered his lungs. Mira refused to sign for the immediate surgery that was required. For a week, the baby survived on fluids provided intravenously. Then, the hospital served Mira an ultimatum: authorise surgery or take the baby home. She chose the latter. Still unable to suckle and deprived of his IV supply, the baby died. For three years after that, Mira battled depression. 'All this was avoidable had the law permitted "late abortion"', says her gynaecologist.

A similar case in the US, known as the Baby Doe controversy, triggered a national debate on the issue of abortion and euthanasia. Born in 1982 with Down's syndrome and a blocked oesophagus, the child at issue in that controversy required immediate corrective surgery to save his life. Although the surgery would have been both routine and low risk, the physicians treating the infant at the hospital disagreed about the proper course of action. One group suggested immediate surgery. The other suggested that the infant receive no treatment and be allowed to die. After a short deliberation, the child's parents chose the latter course. They reasoned that people with Down's syndrome could not achieve a 'minimally acceptable quality of life' and that, therefore, death would be best for the infant, their two other children, and the family as a whole (Muller 2009).

Reflecting upon the above situations, Asch and Fine (1986) have analysed the issue from the perspective of both disability rights and reproductive rights. They argue that women have the right to abortion for any reason they deem appropriate. Newborns with disabilities too have the right to medical treatment whether or not their parent(s) wish them to be treated. Both rights are unequivocal, consistent and currently protected by statute, at least in the US. Both sets of rights are, however, under severe attack and together they have been juxtaposed as contradictory. The authors argue that it is essential to preserve both sets of rights. On the one hand, women have won the right to abortion as a part of the right to control their bodies. On the other hand, the issue of the foetus' rights within a woman's body, particularly if the foetus has a disability, and its right to medical treatment soon after birth, is still debated.

The origin of the debate gained prominence with the case of the Baby Doe. The reasons used to justify denial of medical treatment to such infants have been the reasons given by people who believe that living with a disability is either not worth living, too costly to the family, or too costly to the rest of the non-disabled society. Such prejudice and discrimination against people with disabilities is no surprise. Recognising that parents who are grief-stricken, shocked and anxious may seek to end the lives of their 'imperfect' infants, Asch and Fine argue that they should be counselled, educated and told that the child will receive treatment whether or not the parent(s) agree. The authors are of the firm opinion that the state should work towards a policy in which the government picks up the medical expenses associated with such treatment, where parents are given extensive information about what it means to have a disability, and should be assured of informed consent if they wish to put up their child for adoption or foster care. They believe that the government has a major responsibility for assisting the child with a disability and their families throughout life (Asch and Fine 1986).

Similar ethical choices that had to be made in some cases exist in the narratives. In one case, a form of euthanasia seemed to be endorsed by the doctors themselves. Soon after the child was born, the doctor told the father that the child would be severely disabled physically and, further, suggested to him that since he was a young man and could have more children who would be normal, carrying a burden for an entire lifetime made no sense. The doctor was willing to help give an injection to the child that would 'finish him off'. The father was taken aback by this suggestion and told the doctor no matter what the condition of the child, it was *his* child, and he certainly did not want to 'eliminate' him.

In another case, the mother who was a widow belonging to a low-income family had severe financial problems apart from the practical difficulties in looking after the child with disability. Seeing her condition, her neighbours suggested that she should either abandon the child or stop feeding the baby and it would gradually wither away. The mother could not bear these comments and felt guilty about having borne such a child. However, it was the support of her older two children and an organisation that gave her the strength and confidence to fight these comments, and she is thankful that she did not listen to the neighbours.

In this context, a study by the feminist Rayna Rapp (2000), which begins with her own account of choosing to terminate a pregnancy where the unborn child was diagnosed as having Down's syndrome, is significant. Her personal decision led Rapp to study families that tested for abnormalities and then chose to either terminate or continue with the pregnancy. She found that the decision to continue with the pregnancy or not was determined by class and race location: Families that were still rooted in strong familial ties more often than individuated nuclear families chose to continue with the pregnancy. This tells us something about the cultural context of handling disability and notions of difference.

Stowe et al. (2006) sum up the complex debates around some of the themes raised. They argue that in the past half-century, medical advances in prenatal and neonatal care have recast the moral landscape at the edge of life, death and disability. Therefore, a cautious approach to new reproductive technologies needs to be taken to ensure that the possibilities of present and future eugenic practices are not masked as science. With rapid advances in reproductive technologies, the availability of emerging prenatal genetic testing now allows for the detection of genetic abnormalities, among embryos or in the foetus, which would have previously gone undetected.

On the one hand, the new genetic screening technologies make it possible to discern characteristics of the unborn and abort it on the basis of prenatal disability; on the other hand, improvements in neonatal care allow doctors to save newborns previously beyond hope, many of whom possess disabilities that can be treated but cannot be cured. These advances have thrust intractable questions upon parents, prospective parents and the law. The use of such technology has generally been presented as unquestionable; however, it has raised a myriad of ethical, medical and legal dilemmas for all those involved. When is it acceptable to have an abortion on the basis of prenatal disability? When is it acceptable to refuse life-saving treatment on the basis of neonatal disability? More broadly, when should parents and prospective parents choose death rather than nascent life with a disability (Stowe et al. 2006)? There are no definitive answers.

THE POLITICAL ECONOMY OF DISABILITY

The attempt in this study has been not to leave the narratives merely as qualitative insights into the lives and experiences of the disabled and their parents. On the contrary, this study has tried to argue that while they are derived from a small sample from the urban and rural areas, with families belonging to upper, middle and lower income groups, a range of issues emerge that point to problems faced by families across income groups, but particularly by lower income groups. The issue would be multiplied several fold in the light of the quantum and variety of disabilities that are evident from the Census and NSS data. These data show the characteristics, distribution and health-seeking behaviour of the people. The narratives reveal a thin layer of the scenario prevalent in urban and rural areas respectively that leads one to visualise what the condition would be in the rest of the country. The narratives highlight that there are various categories of populations such as agricultural workers, daily wagers, domestic workers and migrant workers who do not even have the most basic facilities for diagnosis and information about disability.

Overall the narratives highlight the fact that lifelong caregiving and its consequences are at the heart of the experience of families that have children with CP. The narratives also show that the stresses can be unbearable without external support, especially from the state. In a similar way to studies that have shown the relationship between poverty and disability, the narratives too indicate that the intensity of suffering increases as one goes down the class gradient. In a study by Sen cited in Harriss-White (1999, 140), the relationship between poverty (economic disability), 'weakness' (social disability) and the incidence of medical disability has been studied.

Sen has found that 'simultaneous deprivation' is further compounded by a syndrome composed of ideological reinforcement, punitive experience and psychological extinction. This syndrome sets up barriers against participation of all types of disabled people, especially the mentally disabled and girls, in social development. Similarly, another study based on a census of three villages in northern Tamil Nadu, working with people's own definition of chronically sick and disabled household members, showed a positive association between disability and poverty (Harriss-White 1999, 141).

D. Mohan points out that there is also the argument of an inverse relation between income poverty and the prevalence of disability on the grounds that mortality from disability is greatest among the poor. There is evidence of a disability transition during which disabilities due to malnutrition and infectious/contagious disease are eradicated. This disability transition is more than offset by reduced mortality rates, survival of paraplegics and quadriplegics and increases in disabilities due to trauma and old age, such that the total incidence of disability increases (Harriss-White 1999, 142).

Helander has remarked on the existence of international evidence for the aforementioned inverse relationship (Harriss-White 1999, 142). According to Harriss-White, the international evidence of the inverse relationship even in developed countries, however, is no excuse for non-interventionism in the lives of the disabled poor in India because raised levels of mortality clearly result from the economic incapacity of poor families to sustain the lives of disabled members (Harriss-White 1999, 142).

Another aspect of the relationship between poverty and disability is revealed by the NSS data. NSS data show that especially in rural areas the major reason for 'not taking treatment' is that the treatment is too expensive. It is only a small percentage of persons who were not aware of the availability of treatment and, therefore, did not access treatment. The issue of the treatment being too expensive is not just about the expense involved in acquiring the aids or the appliances, but is also about the issue of incidental costs. For instance, even in this study, the rehabilitation of the disabled in rural and urban areas, it was found that although specialist services in government hospitals were given free of cost, incidental expenses such as transport, boarding and lodging, and loss of daily wages took a toll on family income and, therefore, hampered accessing medical intervention. Hence, studies do suggest a relation between poverty and disability.

Another factor revealed by the narratives is that the experience of disability is not merely an individual's experience. If one were to take the disability problem as the suffering of an individual person or a single family, then the related issues and consequent suffering could be alleviated with the help of social work and psychology, the two disciplines which have been associated with disability for a long time. It is at this level that the NGOs' response to help the disabled individual and the family members comes in.

The NGOs can provide psychological and emotional support, along with inputs in training the family to handle the person with disability. However, if one takes cognisance of the fact that suffering is real from a population perspective, and that it is exacerbated by the lack of services and support to the lifelong caring that is required in the case of the disabled, then data show the need for looking at agencies which can deal with disability at the level of the wider population. This is where the state needs to come in.

One of the important ways through which the state can reach out to the disabled and their families is the health service. Rehabilitation is one of the aims, as well as services of primary health care along with prevention, cure and the promotion of health. Hence, basic services pertaining to diagnosis and information regarding disability should be provided at the primary level rather than at the secondary or tertiary level. In a study by Burrett, the lack of referral services for the disabled at the district level resulted in over 50 per cent of the cases dropping out from the treatment process because of the problems of time, distance and money involved to go to the city hospital (Baru 1989).

Poor socio-economic conditions proved to be yet another constraint, especially for families who were daily wage earners. Extending the case further, the daily wage earners not only lose one day's wages but many days because they would have to make repeated trips to the hospital since the assessment, provision of aids or appliances and continued monitoring of the aids would not be done in one day. In such families, a child with disability is not a priority in the light of more pressing burdens, as shown by Burrett (Baru 1989). Hence, district level health services should be provided at the primary level to facilitate access and reach out to the felt needs of the people. These studies reveal the substantive issues in the health-seeking behaviour of the persons interviewed. This is contrary to the commonly held belief that people do not seek treatment for the disabled because they resort to beliefs such as *karma* or *kismet*.

There is a noticeable degree of discomfort attached to the use of the term burden when used in the context of caregiving. The mixed or ambivalent feelings towards caregiving being a burden seems to imply that the person is a burden and, therefore, not normal. However, it should be understood that till such time as an adequate social and economic support system is provided by the state, the condition and life of a person with disability is also going to be viewed in terms of misery. This view is compounded by the attitude and stereotype of disabled people as burdensome.

It is important to bear in mind that arguing for providing services at the primary level is not to make a case for the medicalised model of disability. However, there is a justification to make a demand for a more accessible system for all sections of society since it is known that access to requisite services is related, at the moment, to the class to which the person with disability belongs. The areas in which the state can intervene at the primary level are: providing basic technology for diagnosis, information and prognosis; formulating a treatment plan (not only a medical plan but a course of action that provides requisite aids and appliances); and establishing a referral system similar to the one for communicable diseases.

Caring is an important component of any health service system, and is not just a need of the person or family of the disabled. In the course of the shifts in public health, viewing the body in mechanical terms has under-emphasised the role or aspects of medical tasks other than just curing. The caring, or palliative aspect, tends to get lost as the body is split into different body systems that need specialists to deal with each of them. As a consequence, 'caring' is accorded a low to negligible priority with regard to time and resources. It is at this level that the NGOs can have a collaborative role with the state in terms of contributing their expertise and skills. Therefore, it is important to have health services that are innovative so that facilities for the disabled have a far greater scope.

Thus, we can see that public health has a role to play in the area of disability. This is similar to the case of any communicable disease, as the NSS data provides epidemiological evidence for it. The health-seeking behaviour of people can be assessed too. The fact that there are different needs involved is to be recognised. Since public health has a holistic perspective towards human life, it has to offer the services right from the primary level onwards. Thus, while psychological and social support may not necessarily be provided by the system, it should at least ensure that all the other aspects of disability are addressed in a tangible way.

Apart from the medical, psychological and social needs of the person with disability and their family, the educational, vocational and employment needs are equally important. The narratives highlight the absence of any kind of support measures from the state for all degrees of disability and brings out the hopelessness of the situation. This situation applies in varied degrees across regions and across class. One other major area where the state can intervene is in terms of providing insurance or social security. This would be of significant help because such a measure would go a long way in not just helping the person with disability but the family too.

Therefore, while planning for a meaningful intervention it is important to recognise various emotional, psychological, social and medical needs along with an educational, vocational and employment component. But far from formulating measures to respond to the needs of the disabled, various ministries involved in dealing with issues such as health, education or employment for the disabled are adopting a fragmented approach to framing policies. This is the most important barrier operating in the field of disability. A holistic approach would be able to address all the needs of the disabled outlined earlier: instead a segregation model, which is really a charity model, still prevails.

The argument made here is not just for a statist intervention—because certain functions, perhaps, require the NGOs' skills and expertise that can provide the personal touch. Nonetheless, it is more than clear that the NGO cannot supplant the state. The frustration experienced and expressed by the persons in the narratives directed towards the NGOs is partly because the state has abdicated its responsibilities. Instead, the state neglects its role as the protector of people's rights as part of an integrated perspective operating in the larger system. At the same time, the demand for public intervention does not wipe out the possibilities of or the spaces for private response in many areas. In order to join social and health policy, social services along with health services, and social theory together with health science perspectives must have a place in policy formulation.

Given the dire need for care, services, resources and the right to equal opportunities, there is a need for creative and sympathetic interaction and action on the part of both the state and society, not an artificial dichotomisation of the two arenas.

BEYOND INDIVIDUAL SUFFERING

The literature on disability, and the narratives of parents, professionals and disabled activists that form the basis of this study, suggest that suffering is actually prevalent in the lives of the disabled and those close to them. The accounts of frustration, anger and anguish experienced by the young adolescent person with disability whose helplessness has been invisibilised by society, along with discussions about issues of faith, the importance of family support and the adverse effects of the lack of state support are all indicators of the social suffering undergone by the person with disability as well as the families at various stages in their lives.

Suffering

All the narratives highlight that no matter what the social and economic class of the family, suffering is prevalent across all of them. It is only the level and amount of suffering experienced that is relative. A well-off family may be able to afford state of the art technology for assistive devices, hire help to look after the person and have access to other facilities to make life apparently smooth. Regardless, at the end of the day they still have to face a situation that is similar to the daily struggles of their lower income counterparts, which is dealing with a persons with disability.

While some parents have resources or build them internally to strengthen their own resilience to cope with adversity, there are some who cannot make it through. Many develop chronic health problems due to the ongoing stress, while some develop psychosomatic problems, and in one case the socio-economic situation as well as the child's disability was so overwhelming for the mother that she decided to end her life as well as that of the child, as described in Chapter 7.

While disability is a medical condition it is also a condition that requires caring. Both conditions are lifelong, which is an integral aspect of suffering. Although people deal with disability at an individual level, the suffering is not only an individual experience but has a strong social component to it. There is an absence of basic facilities that would help in reducing the disability factor, and enhance sorely needed self-help skills. These resources that include medical knowledge, access to services, acquiring aids and appliances, and developing skills for training, all affect the quality of life of the disabled. Apart from the fact that the social, psychological, educational and employment possibilities that the disabled have a right to, are not enhanced, these deprivations and the need for 'care' in the widest sense of the term create enormous suffering for those affected by disability.

Disability is socially constructed. However, what is important to note is that even the acknowledgement that disability is socially constructed has not led to the recognition that the 'social' construction is tilted in a certain direction: It is still seen primarily as an issue that is of an 'individual' rather than of a 'social' concern. This limited way of seeing the social construction of disability is a discourse shared by policy-makers, professionals, those advocating CBR and most of the disabled rights activists.

This way of thinking about the 'social' construction of disability may be attributed to the fact that stigma and charity are still strong underlying reasons that creep into the way disability continues to be constructed even today. However, stigma is not the only cause of suffering as has been revealed by the studies and narratives examined in this work. The political economy is a crucial aspect of the way suffering is experienced by those affected by disability. Despair is a dominant motif in the lives of the disabled poor and their families. For the families of the disabled, the intense struggle to care for the disabled is compounded by the lack of facilities of any kind as they put in great effort to earn enough to fulfil their subsistence needs.

Even for those who are better off, the wider political economy determines the way disability is perceived. Inclusion is necessary in every aspect of society—in the area of education, employment or just in neighbourhood activities. There is a need to sensitise society towards the inclusion of the disabled and the possibility of disability in their own lives. For example, when a person becomes disabled in old age, especially a man, his family or others around do not undervalue him because he is judged by the fact that at one time he was a productive individual. From this we can see that the value of labour potential, or its absence, is a structural factor in the current view of the disabled. The fact that an old man who is disabled is not marginalised, as a child with disability would be from the beginning of its life, tells us something about the need to rethink the relationship between the individual and the social. We also need to rethink the relationship between disability and society, and also between disability and the state, both of which reflect the political economy.

As of now, disability continues to be seen as a 'burden', which must be borne by the family with fortitude and patience; disability is still constructed as a situation where 'suffering' is inevitable. The most common way of dealing with pain and suffering is to be tough and bear it all since all those who are involved with disability in India, as parents, as disabled, as professionals and as disability activists, are still trying to formulate their understanding of the wider context in which disability needs to be located. The relationship between the state, society and family in the context of disability is also yet to be formulated.

Just as I was at the tail end of the writing of this work, I came across three instances which once again took me back to the issues raised in the narratives: those of caregiving and suffering and its inevitability in the lives of those who experience disability. I was struck by how the narratives I had consciously collected by seeking families out were constantly being expanded by stray conversations I or my close friends had with their friends or acquaintances. It was almost as if everyone had a story about a family that had a child with CP.

One friend recounted the case of a family that had three CP girls born in the 1960s, two of whom had died in their early years. One of the girls had survived and been cared for by her mother who had given up a career to do so. The surviving child had not been through any training at a special school of sorts, even though such schools had begun to come up in the early 1970s, and despite the fact that the family was from a middle-class background. Both mother and daughter had lived out their lives in isolation from the rest of the world and had borne their sufferings with fortitude—or so it would seem.

Another story that I stumbled upon was from a friend who shared a long car ride with an acquaintance, a man in his late 40s, who was dropping her home. A casual question about whether the acquaintance had siblings revealed this unexpected account:

> The parents of the narrator were from a middle class background and were married in the early 1960s. The father was posted mainly in small towns in North India and was transferred frequently. Their first child, a girl, was born with CP. Shocked by this unexpected turn of events, and unable to cope with a situation where no medical facilities or professional opinion that might lead the parents to know what they could do existed—there were no special schools in those days and no knowledge of them in the small towns—the parents gave away the child to an institutional home to be cared for.
>
> They then had a second child; again it was a girl and she too had CP. Full of dilemmas on what to do with her, they were in a sense hampered by the reactions they had from friends and relatives who told them that the second child too was born with CP because the parents had abandoned the first child. This was a message of sorts that they must not do the same again because then they would never have a normal child. And so the baby stayed with the parents and the mother cared for her.
>
> A few years later, the parents had a third child. This time the baby was a boy and he was normal. As he grew up, he was the centre of the parent's attention. They hoped that he would do well—a normal middle-class aspiration for most of the Indians. The brother and sister had something of a sibling relationship as he helped to carry his sister around. But aspirations for a good education and then a good career were hampered by the presence of a growing young disabled woman who required considerable care and attention.

Finally, the family decided to leave the daughter in another institution. This institution is well reputed for its care and humane attitude to those left in their care. The brother had many memories of his sister but, pushing his memories away, went on to build a life for himself and support his parents in their old age. Some years after giving the second daughter away the family tried to track down the two sisters who had been left to the custody of others, but could not do so as no decisive information was forthcoming.

Was it right for the family to do what they did is still a question that haunts them. They are also troubled by the memories of the children given away. Whatever decisions the families of those with CP children take, grief and suffering seem inevitable.

The latest incident that I came across was a report in the newspaper: The account described a plea for euthanasia by a 34-year-old mother belonging to a poor family. She had to care for her 14-year-old daughter Madhumita who had severe CP. She said she could not remain a mere witness to the sufferings of her daughter; the girl could not communicate with anyone: 'Her only mode of expression is crying', said the mother. The family had taken Madhumita to a special school in Tiruchy, but they had refused to admit her; they also went to hospitals in Thanjavur, Erode and Tiruchy to try and give her special training. It was all in vain. The plea for euthanasia is based on the ground that the parents do not have sufficient means to care for her: The mother needs to go to work since the father's income is not sufficient to feed the family; worrying about the girl's future, the mother has filed a plea for euthanasia.[1]

These instances, even as I close my work, bring to the fore what Marta Russell said in an incisive piece of writing reflecting the understanding of a disabled woman. Her piece was entitled 'The Political

---

[1] Should this Mother's Euthanasia Plea be Granted for her Daughter? https://www.idiva.com/news-relationships/should-this-mothers-euthanasia-plea-be-granted-for-her-daughter/13768 (last accessed on 7 June 2018).

Economy Affects Us All' (Russell 1998). Perhaps we can add 'whether we recognise it or not'. And until then:

> Across our countryside, shrouded from our collective view and conscience people with disability and their care-givers somehow are living out their lives, surviving, but only just, most often on the precipice of dark despair. It is probably only when they organise into a social and political collective voice and assertion that an uncaring state and society will finally be forced to act. (Mander 2002)

APPENDIX

INTERVIEWS WERE CONDUCTED WITH THE FOLLOWING PERSONS WORKING IN OR INVOLVED WITH THE DISABILITY SECTOR

Anita Ghai, University of Delhi, Delhi (Professor, Psychologist and Disability Rights Activist)

Anuradha Naidu, Council for Advancement of People's Action and Rural Technology (CAPART), Delhi (professional and Head of the Disability Unit)

Javed Abidi, National Centre for Promotion of Employment for Disabled Persons (NCPEDP), Delhi (Director and Disability Rights activist)

K.R. Rajendra, Leonard Cheshire International, Bangalore (Director)

Poonam Natarajan, Vidya Sagar, Chennai (Parent, Professional and Director)

Radhika Menon, University of Delhi, Delhi (Assistant Professor and Professional)

Rama Chari, working in NCPEDP, Delhi

Ranjana Pandey, Jan Madhyam, Delhi (Director)

Renu Singh, Spastics Society of Northern India (SSNI), Delhi (Professional and Director)

Shanti Auluck, Muskaan, Delhi (Professor, Psychologist and Director)

BIBLIOGRAPHY

Abbot, P., and R. Sapsford. *Community Care for Mentally Handicapped Children*. Milton Keynes: Open University Press, 1987.

Ablon, J. '"The Elephant Man" as "Self" and "Other": The Psycho-social Costs of a Misdiagnosis'. *Social Science and Medicine* 40, no. 11 (1995): 1481–89.

Abrams, P. *Historical Sociology*. London: Open Books, 1982.

Albrecht, G. L. 'Cross National Rehabilitation Policies: A Critical Assessment'. In *Cross National Rehabilitation Policies: A Sociological Perspective*, edited by G. L. Albrecht. London: SAGE, 1981.

Albrecht, G. L., and J. A. Levy. 'Constructing Disabilities as Social Problems'. In *Cross National Rehabilitation Policies: A Sociological Perspective*, edited by G. L. Albrecht. London: SAGE, 1981.

Allen, D. 'Creating a Public Health Focus on Disability'. Paper presented at National Conference on Disability and Health: Building Bridges for Science and Consumers, Texas, 1998.

Alur, M. *Invisible Children: A Study of Policy Exclusion*. Delhi: Viva Books, 2003.

Asch, A., and M. Fine. 'Shared Dreams: A Left Perspective on Disability Rights and Reproductive Rights'. In *Women with Disabilities: Essays in Psychology, Culture and Politics*, edited by M. Fine and A. Asch. Philadelphia, PA: Temple University Press, 1986.

Banerji, D. *Health and Family Planning Services in India: An Epidemiological, Sociocultural and Political Analysis and a Perspective*. New Delhi: Lok Paksh, 1985.

Baquer, A. *Disability: Challenges and Responses*. New Delhi: Concerned Action Now, 1994.

———. *Disabled, Disablement, Disabilism*. New Delhi: Voluntary Health Association of India, 1994.

———. *Disability: Challenges vs. Responses*. 1997. Available at www.healthlibrary.com (accessed on 13 April 2018).

Barnes, C., G. Mercer, and T. Shakespeare. *Exploring Disability: A Sociological Introduction*. Cambridge: Polity Press, 1999.

Barnes, M. *Care, Communities and Citizens*. London: Longman, 1997.

Baru, R. 'Rehabilitation of Child with Disability: Lessons from Two Community Projects'. *Indian Journal of Social Work* 50 (1989): 227–233.

Becker, G., Y. Beyene, and P. Ken. 'Health, Welfare Reform, and Narratives of Uncertainty among Cambodian Refugees'. *Culture, Medicine, and Psychiatry* 24, no. 2 (2000): 139–163.

Berube, M. *Life as We Know It: A Father, a Family and an Exceptional Child*. New York, NY: Vintage, 1998.

Brisenden, S. 'Independent Living and the Medical Model of Disability'. *Disability, Handicap and Society* 1, no. 2 (1986): 173–78.

Burton, M. 'Understanding Mental Health Services: Theory and Practice'. *Critical Social Policy* 3, no. 7 (1983): 54–74.

Cameron, D. David Cameron: The Five Lessons I Learned as Father of Disabled Child—and Intend to Put into Practice. Independent, 2009. Available at http://www.independent.co.uk/news/uk/politics/david-cameron-the-five-lessons-i-learned-as-father-of-disabled-child-ndash-and-intend-to-put-into-practice-1748274.html (accessed on 13 April 2018).

Chakravarti, U. 'Is Suffering Inevitable: State, Society and Disability'. Unpublished MPhil Thesis, Centre of Community Health and Social Medicine, Jawaharlal Nehru University, 2002.

Chatterjee, P. 'Approaches to the Welfare State'. 1997. Available at www.naswpress.org (accessed on 13 April 2018).

Chib, M. *One Little Finger*. New Delhi: SAGE, 2011a.

———. I'm Single Because of My Body. *The Times of India*, 2011b. Available at http://articles.timesofindia.indiatimes.com/2011-09-20/man-woman/30179999_1_disabled-people-disabled-activists-disabled-women (accessed on 13 April 2018).

Cohen L. 'Where It Hurts: Indian Material for an Ethics of Organ Transplantation'. *Daedalus* 128, no. 4 (1999): 135–165.

CommunityCare. Cameron Writes to Mother of Disabled Child Who Can't Cope. 2011. Available at http://www.communitycare.co.uk/2011/01/20/cameron-writes-to-mother-of-disabled-child-who-cant-cope/ (accessed on 13 April 2018).

Conrad, P., and J. Schneider. *Deviance and Medicalization: From Badness to Sickness*. St. Louis, MA: Mosby, 1980.

Crichton, A. 'Development of Rehabilitation Policies in Britain, Canada and Australia: A Comparison'. In *Cross National Rehabilitation Policies: A Sociological Perspective*, edited by G. L. Albrecht. London: SAGE, 1981.

Curtis, S., N. Petukhova, G. Sezonova, and N. Netsenko. 'Caught in the "Traps of Managed Competition?" Examples of Russian Health Care Reforms from St. Petersburg and the Leningrad Region'. *International Journal of Health Services* 27, no. 4 (1997): 661–86.

Dalal, A. K. 'CBR in Action—Some Reflections from the Sirathu Project'. *Asia Pacific Disability Rehabilitation Journal* 9, no. 1 (1998): 96–105.

Dalley, G. *Ideologies of Caring: Rethinking Community and Collectivism*. London: Macmillan, 1988.
Daly, M., & K. Rake. *Gender and the Welfare State: Care, Work and Welfare in Europe and the USA*. Cambridge: Polity Press, 2003.
Du Boff, R. B. 'The Welfare State, Pensions, Privatization: The Case of Social Security in the United States'. *International Journal of Health Services* 30, no. 1 (1997): 1–23.
Eriksen, T. R., and H. M. Dahl. 'Dilemmas of Care in the Nordic Welfare State'. 2005. Available at www.ashgate.com
Farmer, P. 'On Suffering and Structural Violence: A View from Below'. In *Social Suffering*, edited by A. Kleinman, V. Das and M. M. Lock. Berkeley, CA: University of California Press, 1997.
George, V., and P. Wilding. *Ideology and Social Welfare*. London: Routledge & Kegan Paul, 1985.
Ghai, A. 'Refocusing on the Child with Disability', 2001. Available at www.leeds.ac.uk/disability-studies (accessed on 13 April 2018).
———. *(Dis)Embodied Form: Issues of Disabled Women*. Delhi: Shakti Books, 2003.
Giddens, A. *Sociology*. Cambridge: Polity Press, 1989.
Gilson, L., P. D. Sen, S. Mohammed, and P. Mujinja. 'The Potential of Health Sector Non-governmental Organizations: Policy Options'. *Health Policy and Planning* 9, no. 1 (1994): 14–24.
Goffman, E. *Asylums: Essays on the Social Situation of Mental Patients and Other Inmates*. Chicago, IL: Aldine Publishing Company, 1976.
Goldin, C. S., and J. Scheer. 'Murphy's Contributions to Disability Studies: An Inquiry into Ourselves'. *Social Science and Medicine* 40, no. 11 (1995): 1443–45.
Gough, I. *The Political Economy of the Welfare State*. London: Macmillan, 1979.
Government of India. The Persons with Disabilities (Equal Opportunities, Protection of Rights and Full Participation) Act 1995, Parliament of India, New Delhi, 1995.
———. Census of India. New Delhi: Government of India, 1981.
———. Census of India. New Delhi: Registrar General and Census Commissioner, Government of India, 2001.
Guterman, L. Choosing Eugenics: How Far Will Nations Go to Eliminate a Genetic Disease? *Chronicle of Higher Education* 9, no. 34 (2003): A22–A26.
Harriss-White, B. 'On to a Loser: Disability in India'. In *Illfare in India: Essays on India's Social Sector in Honour of S. Guhan*, edited by B. Harriss-White and S. Subramaniam. New Delhi: SAGE, 1999.
Should this mother's euthanasia plea be granted for her daughter? Available at https://www.idiva.com/news-relationships/should-this-mothers-euthanasia-plea-be-granted-for-her-daughter/13768 (accessed on 4 July 2012).
Jayal, N. G. 'The Gentle Leviathan: Welfare and the Indian State'. *Social Scientist* 22, no. 9–12 (1994): 18–26.
Jeffery, R., and N. Singal. 'Measuring Disability in India'. *Economic & Political Weekly* 43, no. 12 & 13 (2008): 22–24.

Johansson, S. 'Women's Paradise Lost? Care in the Quasi-markets in Sweden'. Available at http://www.ashgate.com/pdf/SamplePages/DilemmasofCareIntro.pdf

Jones, G. 'Health Care Access and Utilisation Patterns of Persons with Severe Activity Limitations'. Paper presented at National Conference on Disability and Health: Building Bridges for Science and Consumers, Texas, 1998.

Jones, K., and A. Tilotson. *The Adult Population of Epileptic Colonies*. London: British Epilepsy Association and International Bureau for Epilepsy, 1965.

Kittay, E. F. *Love's Labour: Essays on Women, Equality and Dependency*. New York: Routledge, 1998.

Kleinman, A. *Writing at the Margin: Discourse Between Anthropology and Medicine*. Berkley: University of California Press, 1995.

Kleinman, A., V. Das, and M. Lock, eds. *Social Suffering*. New Delhi: Oxford University Press, 1997.

Kleinman, A., W. Z. Wang, S. C. Li, X. M. Cheng, X. Y. Dai, K. T. Li, and J. Kleinman. 'The Social Course of Epilepsy: Chronic Illness as Social Experience in Interior China'. *Social Science and Medicine* 40, no. 10 (1995): 19–30.

Kolberg, J. E. 'Conceptions of Social Disability'. In *Cross National Rehabilitation Policies: A Sociological Perspective*, edited by G. L. Albrecht. London: SAGE, 1981.

Langan, M., ed. *Welfare: Needs, Rights and Risks*. London: Routledge, 1998.

Leichter, H. M. *A Comparative Approach to Policy Analysis: Health Care Policy in Four Nations*. Cambridge: Cambridge University Press, 1979.

Madison, B. Q. *Social Welfare in the Soviet Union*. Stanford: Stanford University Press, 1968.

Mander, H. 'At the Precipice of Despair'. *Frontline*, 2 August 2002.

Marteau, T. M., and H. Drake. 'Attributions for Disability: The Influence of Genetic Screening'. *Social Science and Medicine* 40, no. 8 (1995): 1127–32.

Marshall, T. H. *Class, Citizenship and Social Development*. Chicago, IL: University of Chicago Press, 1964.

Mitra, S., and U. Sambamoorthi. 'Disability Estimates in India: What the Census and NSS Tell Us'. *Economic & Political Weekly* 41, no. 38 (2006): 23–29.

Mont, D. Measuring Disability Prevalence, SP Discussion Paper No. 0706, The World Bank, 2007. Available at http://siteresources.worldbank.org/DISABILITY/Resources/Data/MontPrevalence.pdf (last accessed on 7 June 2018).

Muller, J. 'The New Parenthood and the Old Ambivalence about Disability: Baby Doe, Prenatal Testing, and Disability Rights'. Student Prize Paper, Yale Law School, Connecticut, 2009.

Navarro, V. 'The Political Economy of the Welfare State in Developed Capitalist Countries'. *International Journal of Health Services* 29, no. 1 (1999): 1–50.

National Sample Survey Organisation (NSSO). 'Persons with Disability in India'. Report No. 485. New Delhi: Government of India, 2002.

———. 36th Round, July–December, Government of India, 1981.

———. 47th Round, July–December, Government of India, 1991.

Nussbaum, M. 'Disabled Lives: Who Cares?' *New York Review of Books* 48, no. 1 (2001): 34–37.

Oliver, M. *The Politics of Disablement: A Sociological Approach*. New York, NY: St. Martin's Press, 1990.

Oliver, M. *Understanding Disability: From Theory to Practice*. London: Macmillan, 1996.

Pardo, P. 'Portraits of Pity or Possibility? Images of People with Disability from Around the World'. *Disability Information Network*, 2000.

Parker, R. 'A Historical Background'. In *Residential Care: The Research Reviewed*, edited by I. Sinclair. London: Her Majesty's Stationery Office, 1988.

Pasternak, J. 'An Analysis of Social Perceptions of Epilepsy: Increasing Rationalisation as Seen Through the Theories of Comte and Weber'. *Social Science and Medicine* 15E, no. 3 (1981): 223–29.

Pessagno., A. Richard, 'Grief, Loss and Bereavement'. Available at www.nursing-ceu.com (last accessed in 2006).

Phillips, S. D. '"There Are No Invalids in the USSR!": A Missing Soviet Chapter in the New Disability History'. *Disability Studies Quarterly* 29, no. 3 (2009): 1–35.

Preston P. 'Mother Father Deaf: The Heritage of Difference'. *Social Science and Medicine* 40, no. 11 (1995): 1461–67.

Qadeer, I. 'Health Services System in India: An Expression of Socio-economic Inequalities'. *Social Action* 35, no. 3 (1985): 199–223.

Rapp, R. *Testing Women, Testing the Fetus: The Social Impact of Amniocentesis in America*. New York, NY: Routledge.

Razavi, S., and S. Staab, eds. *Global Variation in the Political and Social Economy of Care*. New York: Routledge, Routledge/UNRISD Research Series on Gender and Development, 2012.

Rosen, G. 'Historical Trends and Future Prospects in Public Health'. In *History and Medical Care: A Symposium of Perspectives*, edited by T. McKeown. London: Nuffield, 1971.

Russell, M. *Beyond Ramps: Disability at the End of the Social Contract*. Monroe, ME: Common Courage Press, 1998.

Russell, M. 'The Political Economy Affects Us Personally'. *Kaleidoscope* no. 38 (1999): 6–13.

Ryan, J., and F. Thomas. *The Politics of Mental Handicap*. Harmondsworth: Penguin, 1980.

Sama—Resource Group for Women and Health. Report on ART and Women. 2006.

Saraga, E., ed. *Embodying the Social: Constructions of Difference*. London: Routledge, 1998.

Scheper-Hughes, N. *Death Without Weeping: The Violence of Everyday Life in Brazil*. Berkeley, CA: University of California Press, 1992.

Shakespeare, T. '2053 AD: After Disability?' 2003. Available at http://www.bbc.co.uk/ouch (accessed on 13 April 2018).

Shourie, A. *Does He Know a Mother's Heart? How Suffering Refutes Religions*. Delhi: Harper Collins, 2011.
Smith, B., and B. Hutchinson. *Gendering Disability*. New Brunswick: Rutgers, 2001.
Stone, D. *The Disabled State*. London: Macmillan. 1985.
Stowe, M. J., H. R. Turnbull III, S. Schrandt, and J. Rack. 'Looking to the Future: Intellectual and Developmental Disabilities in the Genetics Era'. *Journal on Developmental Disabilities* 13, no. 1 (2006): 1–64.
The Hindu. What Women Want: The Ability Debates. 2010. Available at http://www.thehindu.com/life-and-style/metroplus/article420517.ece (accessed on 13 April 2018).
———. Live Like It's Heaven on Earth. 2003. Available at http://www.hindu.com/thehindu/mp/2003/02/25/stories/2003022500060300.htm (accessed on 13 April 2018).
The Times of India. There's Something About Merry. 2010. Available at http://articles.timesofindia.indiatimes.com/2010-01-02/people/28124047_1_autistic-children-neeraj-autistic-son (accessed on 13 April 2018).
The World Bank. People with Disabilities in India: From Commitments to Outcomes, Human Development Unit, South Asia Region, 2007. Available at http://documents.worldbank.org/curated/en/358151468268839622/People-with-disabilities-in-India-from-commitments-to-outcomes (accessed on 13 April 2018).
Thomas, M., and M. J. Thomas. 'Planning for "Community Participation" in CBR'. *Asia Pacific Disability Rehabilitation Journal* 12, no. 1 (2001): 44–51.
Thomas, M. J. 'Community Based Rehabilitation in South Asia: At the Crossroads?' *CBR News*, no. 30 (1999).
Titmuss, R. *Essays on 'The Welfare State'*. London: George Allen & Unwin, 1958.
———. *Commitment to Welfare*. London: George Allen & Unwin, 1968.
Turnbull, D. 'Genetic Counselling: Ethical Mediation of Eugenic Futures?' *Futures*, 32, no. 9–10 (2000): 853–65.
Veeranarayan, K. V. 'Political Economy of State Intervention in Health Care'. *Economic & Political Weekly* 26, no. 42 (1991).
Wadhwa, S. 'Edge of Town'. *Outlook*, 10 August 2001.
Walker, A., and C. K. Wong. 'Rethinking the Western Construction of the Welfare State'. *International Journal of Health Services* 26, no. 1 (1996): 67–92.
Williams, J. *Unbending Gender: Why Family and Work Conflict and What to do About It*. New York, NY: Oxford University Press, 1999.
Wilmot, S. *The Ethics of Community Care*. London: Cassell, 1997.
Westbrook, M. T., V. Legge, and M. Pennay. 'Attitudes Towards Disabilities in a Multicultural Society'. *Social Science and Medicine* 36, no. 5 (1993): 615–23.
World Health Organization and World Bank. *World Report on Disability*. 2011.
Zaidi, S. A. 'NGO Failure and the Need to Bring Back the State'. *Journal of International Development* 11, no. 2 (1999): 259–71.
Zola, I. K. 'Self, Identity and the Naming Question: Reflections on the Language of Disability'. *Social Science and Medicine* 36, no. 2 (1993): 167–73.

INDEX

Abidi, Javed, 150, 156
Able Disabled All People Together (ADAPT), Mumbai, 90–93
able-bodied scoundrels, 173
abortion, 189–197
Action for Ability Development and Inclusion (AADI), New Delhi, 6, 7, 8
Action for Autism, New Delhi, 89, 93–94
adults with disabilities, working experience, 5
aged population, increasing trend in developed countries, 121
All India Institute of Medical Sciences (AIIMS), 91
Alur, Mithu, 89, 90
Anganwadi project, 158
assisted reproductive technologies (ART), 193, 194
Auluck, Shanti, 89, 95
autism, 89

Baby Doe controversy, in US (1982), 194
Balwadi projects, 160
Barua, Merry, 89, 93
behavioural or emotional disorders, 97
Berube, Michael, 23

Cameron, David, 169, 170, 170–171
Canadian Pension Plan of 1965, 180
CAPART, disability movement, 152
care, 119
    definition of, 11
    features of, 11
caregiver health, 129–133
caregiving or caring, concept of, 4, 9, 14–24, 14–24, 120, 120
    formal and informal care, 121
    narratives of, 124–127
    national and international research on aged, 123–124
    organisation of, 122
    perception of disabled persons, 133–134
    social support from family members, 127–129
    types of, 134–135
    unpaid care of mothers, 140–141
    unpaid labour of mother, 135–140
caring about, 16
caring for, 16
caste consciousness, 166
Centre for Special Education (CSE), 91
cerebral palsy (CP) patients, 206
    access to services, 37–42
    act of diagnosis and initial reaction, 31–37

Index

and NGOs role, 68–70
anxiety feeling in, 51–68
child as teacher and support, 82–83
coping with disability, 70–74
cure or miracle, search for, 70–74
faith as succour, 75–76
fathers experience with, 80–82
grief of, 51–68
helplessness, feelings of, 51–68
need for physical space, 45–48
parents with more disable children, 76–78
physical space of house, 45
saviour child, need for, 83–85
siblings as care providers, 85–87
stigma attached with, 48–51
transport, access to, 42–44
who have single mothers, 78–80
Cerebral Palsy Foundation, 10
Chona, Shyama, 90, 98
community-based rehabilitation (CBR), concept of, 159, 165, 167, 168
in India, programmes, 148–150
pre-requisites for, 148
Constitution of India, Article 41 of, 145–146
CP patients
definition of, 10
motor disorders of, 10
rationale for choosing families with, 5–9

Dalal, Ajit, 166
deserving poor, 174
developmental delay, 97
disability/disabled people, 27
and marriage, family and new household, 110–114
as socially constructed, 204
assessment of organizations dealing with, 99–105

awareness among, 150–151
David Cameron appeal to state, 169–170
definition of, 13–14
education and vocational training of person with, 106
individual views of, 10
individualised nature to issue of, 3
movement in India, 151–155
persons with, 3
political economy of, 197–202
requires caring, 204
rights and privileges under Article 41 of Indian constitution, 145–146
seen as burden, 205
social construction of, 204
Disability Rights Group (DRG), 154, 155

epilepsy problem, in China, 27
euthanasia, 189–197

family-based care, 16
Farmer, Paul, 27

Gauthier, David, 21
Ghai, Anita, 153, 155, 157, 162

Harriss-White, Barbara, 14, 14
health welfare policies, 173

inclusive education, for disabled children, 106–109
Industrial Revolution, 174
Integrated Child Development Services (ICDS) programme, 157
International Classification of Impairments, Disabilities and Handicaps (ICIDH), 13
Invalid and Old-age Pensions Act 1941, Australia, 180

Jamia Millia Islamia University, 98
Jan Madhyam, New Delhi, 90, 99

learning disabilities, 97
legitimately poor, 173
love, 16

mental disability, 14, 22, 72
mental retardation, 5, 89, 97
mercantilism, doctrine of, 173
mothers as pioneers, for disabled children, 88–90
Muskaan, New Delhi, 90, 95

Natarajan, Poonam, 89, 154
National Centre for Promotion of Employment for Disabled Persons (NCPEDP), Delhi, 150
National Centre for Promotion of Employment of Disabled Persons (NCPEDP), Delhi, 151, 152
National Sample Survey (NSS), 5
Navarro, Vicente, 176
new reproductive technologies, 189–197
New York Times, 19
NGOs
    criticism of, 187–188
    roles of, 187
non-institutional care, 121
Nussbaum, Martha, 19, 20, 21, 23, 24

Pandey, Ranjana, 90, 98
physical disability, 14, 97
primary goods theory, 22
professional nurse, 134
psychology, 120
public health
    biomedical presence, 4

definition of, 4
interdisciplinary perspective on, 4
PWD Act, 150

Rawls, John, 21, 21
rehabilitation policies, in health care system, 178–188
report of Royal Commission on Compensation and Rehabilitation, 1967, Britain, 182
right to welfare, 165
Rohatgi, Jolly, 98

Sama Resource Group for Women and Health, 193
Sarva Shiksha Abhiyan, 158, 161
Sen, Amartya, 22
Shakespeare, 192
Shourie, Arun, 58, 61, 62, 74, 82, 102
Sick and Disabled Persons Act, 1970, Britain, 181
Sirathu Project, 166
social construction of dependency, 123
social security programme, development of, 176
social suffering, 9, 12
    definition of, 24
    impact of, 24
    in high-income and low-income societies, 25
    inter-subjective experience, implications of, 26
    Western tradition experience, 25
social support, 127–129
social work, 120, 199
social workers, 96, 113
Spastics Society of India, 89

Spastics Society of Northern India (SSNI), 8, 44, 56, 57, 68, 80, 91, 100, 103, 150, 151, 152, 159, 160
status of women (1976), 147
suffering
    as mode of social experience, 59
    as social experience, 25
    disability as, 203–208
    social, 8, 12

Tamana, 90, 98
Together in Education (TIE), 9

Vidya Sagar, Chennai, 89, 95–98
voluntarism, 177

welfare policy, dimensions of, 172
welfare state, 179
welfare state model in India, 162
welfare state
    definition of, 172
    funding and organisation, 176
    in southern European countries, 177
    origin or development of, 172–173, 175
welfare
    camps, 166
    definition of, 171
women and disability, relationship between, 114–118,

ABOUT THE AUTHOR

Upali Chakravarti is Assistant Professor at the Department of Elementary Education, Miranda House, University of Delhi, Delhi. She has done her Masters in Psychology from University of Delhi and PhD from Jawaharlal Nehru University. Her research and teaching interests are in the areas of developmental psychology; education, particularly special and inclusive education; disability studies; and health issues.